CRADLE AND ALL

WOMEN WRITERS

CRADLE AND ALL

ON PREGNANCY AND BIRTH

Edited by
LAURA CHESTER

Faber and Faber
Boston and London

Copyright © 1989 by Laura Chester
The acknowledgments on pp. 261–265 constitute an extension of this copyright notice

Library of Congress Cataloging-in-Publication Data
Cradle and all : women writers on pregnancy and birth / edited by
Laura Chester.
p.   cm.
ISBN 0-571-12989-7 : $12.95
1. Pregnancy—Literary collections.   2. Childbirth—Literary
collections.   3. Motherhood—Literary collections.   4. American
literature—20th century.   5. American literature—Women authors.
I. Chester, Laura.
PS509.P67C7   1989
810.8'0354—dc20   89-11626

Cover design by Jackie Schuman
Printed in the United States of America

This book is dedicated to
Clovis and Ayler,
Loren, Alden, and Joanna.

And for you, I see a big life beginning.
I feel lucky to have been there from the start.

oo oo oo

CONTENTS

ON BEING BORN

THE PAINFUL PARTS

MILK SONGS

FURTHER MOTHERING

oo oo oo

INTRODUCTION

When we are stunned by something completely beautiful, the mind dilates in order to more fully perceive. The natural reaction to this is contraction, for to be opened up is to feel certain pain. The pupils of the eye have this knowledge; they dilate when beholding the beloved. But to love is to be vulnerable to loss. And so it is with childbirth. So it is with writers, who don't turn away, but dare try to set it on the page.

Women seem to have a high threshold for pain as well as a great capacity to behold. It is no surprise that we see in this collection the ability to describe that which is almost indescribable, the most "ordinary miracle" we all share—being born. Our lives are indeed full of ordinary miracles and miseries that can be seen in a linear fashion or as a pattern of concentric circles. It is this series of feminized circles that I wanted to explore through the literary concern of prose and poetry. I wanted to see how women writers would come to the first-hand experience of pregnancy, birth, and early mothering, and how the literalness of that experience might be transformed.

Certainly there are plenty of non-fiction books that can tell a woman what to expect as a fetus develops, from the infinitesimal egg to the body at full term. There are also other collections suitable for shower gifts, but one senses that these books are like good luck talismans, not really meant to be read. I envisioned an anthology with a different scope, with works that didn't shy away from a deeper encounter, that engaged the emotional facts, the woes as well as the wonder.

When I was first pregnant, I was often perplexed by my own ambivalence in contrast to what the birth books told me to expect. I felt as if I were only being allowed to conjure the hazy, euphoric side of mothering. I wanted to believe that birth could be painless—many books told me it could be. Still, I latched onto certain pieces: "Rings," by Daphne Marlatt, and "Birth," by Anaïs Nin, that truly dramatized delivery. It was only through literature that I felt I was getting an honest picture.

Cradle and All begins by looking at the monthly cycle as a time of anticipation and loss, of tension and release. Early on, this rhythm of the lunar egg, building up and letting go, is established in the female psyche. No wonder the moon is our metaphor and that we sometimes resent it, filling and waning, endlessly it seems, until one month everything changes.

What takes place in the nine months of pregnancy *is* awesome. The changes come so fast that the first-time mother is rarely prepared. It is often a difficult time for a writer, having to adjust to the physical pull toward sleep and internal creation when there is also this urgency to record. Intense pain and joy, those brief moments of dilation, are both often lost to us, but here in this collection they are captured. In "Natural Birth" Toi Derricotte gives us these extremes:

> the meat rolls up and moans on the damp table.
> my body is a piece of cotton over another
> woman's body. some other woman, all muscle and
>   nerve, is
> tearing apart and opening under me.

and then:

> why wasn't the room bursting with lilies? why was
> everything the same with them moving so slowly as if
> they were drugged? why were they acting the same
>   when
> suddenly, everything had changed?

In the past, women writers often shied away from the subject of pregnancy and birth, possibly afraid that men might judge it "limited," too focused on the processes of the body. Such fear is a form of self-betrayal, but this anthology documents a real turnaround in the attitude of women writers today.

When I was in college, my poetry teacher told me, "Don't ever get married. You'll end up with children." Never give myself to life? I thought. Would my writing be better if I gave less? Marguerite Duras had this to say in an interview:

> Why discourage women from the colossal swallowing
> up which is the essence of all motherhood, the mad
> love (for it is there, the love of a mother for her child),
> and the madness that maternity represents? For her to
> feel like a man, free from the shackles that it implies?
> That is probably the reason. But if I answer that men
> are sick precisely because of this, because they do not
> have the only opportunity offered a human being to
> experience a bursting of the ego, how would I be
> answered? That it was man who made motherhood the
> monstrous burden it is for sure. But to me the historical

reasons for the burden and drudgery seem the most superficial, because for those there is a remedy. And even if men are responsible for this enslaving form of motherhood, is this enough to condemn maternity itself?

The remedy has been set in motion now that the strict roles of parenting have shifted. The father's participation throughout pregnancy and birth, his bonding with the newborn and care for the infant, has helped widen the boundaries of his own humanity while giving the child a fuller start. But this shifting of the burden is a very slow process, and we are still on middle ground somewhere, only approaching the shared ideal of a balanced life that includes love, writing, children— nurturing the other while caring for the self.

Cradle and All was first intended to be a section in the preceding anthology, *Deep Down: The New Sensual Writing by Women*. I wanted to show how the sensual and the maternal were linked, especially during pregnancy and lactation. Certainly there is no other time when the female body appears so ripe. Images of the Venus of Willandorf arise, with her overwhelming physicality. The pregnant body, once considered unsightly and obese, can now be perceived as sensuously full. Sharon Doubiago writes:

> In the bursting of your coming, muscle, skin, walls,
> the smock untied. I leaned back on my hands,
> my stretched, engorged breasts exposed, laughed,
> entered a strange stream, a sexual
> stream, the ecstacy of time and place, a churning . . .

But while editing *Deep Down*, I could see that *Cradle and All* deserved to be a book with as much diversity as the first. Both of these anthologies bring together some of the best contemporary prose and poetry available in the English language. Though some of the pieces here come close to non-fiction, I feel that all of the work included takes us beyond the status of the mere account, holding language as a primary concern.

I did try to give a full range within each section, showing both the dark and the light sides, but decided to isolate some of the more painful parts that look at miscarriage, infertility, abortion, and the premature infant. Many expectant mothers might not want to carry these images right now, though they might well return to this section later. I do think it's important to empathize with what can and does happen, so that we never gloat over the lives of our healthy children in a way that excludes another woman.

Once you become a mother, you are more keenly aware of the fragility of life and therefore of potential tragedy. Perhaps that is what humanizes the writing here. Mothering actually gives us direct access to the greatest themes in literature—birth, death, loss, love. As Madeline Tiger shows in this short poem, these elements are often intertwined:

> The instant of birth is exquisite.
> Pain and joy are one at this moment.
> Ever after, the dim recollection is
> so sweet that we speak to our children
> with a gratitude they never understand.
> We speak to our parents with a sorrow
> unfamiliar until the day they are dying.

Giving birth is indeed the most remarkable feat a physical body can achieve. We are opened up as at no other time. And when life comes through, the knowledge of that other side is present, sensed. When we witness the newborn, whole and perfect, for the first time, we know that we are connected to "Something Larger," as Sherril Jaffe describes in the closing piece.

The first cradle was within the mother, and children in their metaphorical genius relive the experience over and over through play and rhyme—falling on the hard ground together. "Down will come baby, cradle and all," is an externalization of the process of being born, of coming down to earth. Perhaps writing is also a kind of reenactment, the sweetest form of play the adult mind can achieve. In *Touch to My Tongue*, Daphne Marlatt writes that language is like a living body we enter at birth. "That body of language we speak, our mothertongue. It bears us as we are born into it ..." Coming through the body we go way beyond it, making valid life experience through the context of the word.

NEW BEGINNINGS

oo oo oo

SHERRIL JAFFE

The Baby Laughs _____

Once upon a time there was a little baby waiting on the moon to be born. For a long time it had been watching Ann. It watched Ann and Ben and sighed, for there was not enough love there to bring this babe to earth. And it watched as Ben went away and Ann went about her business, and it drummed its little fingers on the cold surface of the moon, for it was growing impatient.

It had also been watching Abraham. It saw Abraham when he told his girl friend that he didn't want to have any more babies, and it had seen his girl friend say that then he didn't really love her, for if he really loved her he would want to have her baby, and the baby nodded its little head in agreement, for it was made entirely of love, and it knew that this was so. And it watched that woman disappear and Abraham sit alone in his house, unaware that he was being watched.

Then one night when Ann and Abraham had almost despaired of finding true love, God brought them together. Then the babe knew that it wouldn't be long now, and the moon shone a little brighter, for, although many people think that the moon gets its light from reflection, it is love which is the source of all light. And the baby laughed.

oo oo oo

SHERRIL JAFFE

Meanwhile, Back on Earth _____

Meanwhile, back on earth, Abraham was cooking breakfast for Ann. "Say," he said to her as he stirred the eggs, "I've been meaning to ask you. What type of birth control do you use?"

"I use the ovulation method," Ann said.

"The what?" Abraham asked.

"The ovulation method. I figure out when I'm ovulating. A woman is only fertile a few days a month. There's no point in using dangerous drugs or torture devices for the whole month when a woman is only fertile a few days. So I abstain or use a condom when I'm fertile."

"I knew a woman who did it that way. By the phases of the moon. And *she* got pregnant," Abraham said. The toast was starting to burn.

"Well, I don't do it by the moon," Ann said. "I check my temperature and mucus," Ann said. "It's very scientific."

"Well, what if you *do* get pregnant?" Abraham said, taking her in his arms. "That wouldn't be so bad. In fact, it would be wonderful. A little Ann! I can't believe I'm saying this. I never thought I'd feel this way."

"Yes, it *would* be wonderful," Ann said. She couldn't believe he was saying this. She never thought anyone would ever say this to her. "But I don't even know if I can get pregnant," she said. "I've never been pregnant."

"That's the silliest thing I ever heard," Abraham said. "You're the most fertile person I've ever met."

"Do you really think so?" Ann asked.

"Yes, I do," Abraham said. "And I love you. And I want to have your baby."

"Well, we can't try until we're married," Ann said. "I don't even know if I can get pregnant."

"Just give me a chance," the baby said.

oo oo oo

SUMMER BRENNER

Spring Tide _____

There is man-made importance
and there is the lunar egg.

        And in that scarlet orb
almost feathered for conception
there are no illusions of immortality
Only a whiney yolk
to perhaps improbably
further on the species
So precisely every 28 days
we women house a miscellaneous creation
that there in the painful cotton
we are reminded of tides
corn growing in season
ageless labors and ancient orders
fixing us in the tradition of an acorn
        We pass life
and it is garbage
it is graceful waste
it is falling off the roof
as my mother calls it
An opening that bleeds
passing rhythm seasons
musical blood

There is no pretense on the pad
It is biological failure
        The ovary is dutiful not ambitious
It just accidentally fructates the mensual connection
of love for what is life and death

O Isis
my Mississippi
my delta

SHARON OLDS

The Moment _____

When I saw the dark Egyptian stain,
I went down into the house to find you, Mother—
past the grandfather clock, with its huge
ochre moon, past the burnt
sienna woodwork, rubbed and glazed.
I went deeper and deeper down into the
body of the house, down below the
level of the earth. It must have been
the maid's day off, for I found you there
where I had never found you, by the wash tubs,
your hands thrust deep in soapy water,
and above your head, the blazing windows
at the surface of the ground.
You looked up from the iron sink,
a small haggard pretty woman
of 40, one week divorced.
"I've got my period, Mom," I said,
and saw your face abruptly break open and
glow with joy. "Baby," you said,
coming toward me, hands out and
covered with tiny delicate bubbles like seeds.

oo oo oo

SHARON OLDS

The Planned Child _____

I always hated the way they planned me, she
took the cardboards out of his shirts as if
pulling the backbone up out of his body and
made a chart of the month and put her
temperature on it, rising and falling, to
know the day to make me—I always
wanted to have been conceived in heat,
in haste, by mistake, in love, in sex,
not on cardboard, the little X on the
rising line that did not fall again.

But then you were pouring the wine red as the
gritty clay of this earth, or the blood,
grainy with tiny clots, that rides us
into this life, and you said you could tell I had
been a child who was wanted. I took the
wine into my mouth like my mother's blood, as I had
ridden down toward the light with my lips
pressed against the sides of that valve in her body, she was
bearing down and then breathing in the mask and then
bearing down, pressing me out into the
world that was not enough for her without me in it,
not the moon, the sun, the stars, Orion
cartwheeling easily across the dark, not the
earth, the sea, none of it was
enough for her, without me.

SHARON OLDS

Eggs

My daughter has turned against eggs. Age six
to nine, she cooked them herself, getting up
at six to crack the shells, slide the
three yolks into the bowl,
slit them with the whisk, beat them till they hissed
and watch the pan like an incubator as they
firmed, gold. Lately she's gone from
three to two to one and now she
cries she wants to quit eggs.
It gets on her hands, it's slimy, and it's hard
to get all the little things out:
puddles of gluten glisten on the counter
with small, curled shapes floating in their
sexual smear. She moans. It is getting
too close. Next birthday she's ten and then
it's open season, no telling when
the bright, crimson dot appears
like the sign on a fertilized yolk. She has carried
all her eggs in the two baskets
woven into her fine side,
but soon they'll be slipping down gently,
sliding. She grips the counter where the raw
whites jump, and the spiral shapes
signal from the glittering gelatine, and she
wails for her life.

oo oo oo

LYNNE SHARON SCHWARTZ

from: *Rough Strife* _____

When she remarked, much later, that he loved the child
more than he loved her he denied it, naturally. He said he loved Isabel
not more but differently. "Can't you see that? It's so obvious. It's a
different kind of relationship." It was jarring to hear Ivan use words
like "relationship"; it made her doubt certain coveted visions she still
had of him: that he was the noble savage who had approached her
warily, with subtle grace, through the crowd. Or else the reverse, self-
made eighteenth-century man released from the Augustan setting—
balanced and serene, witty and sentimental, yet more attuned to brute
impulse than he cared to acknowledge. But would a primitive or Augustan speak of "relationships"?

In any case, his love for the child didn't appear different in kind to
Caroline. What was so obvious was its sameness. All love was the
same, a desire to gather in and embrace.

Isabel was at her most beautiful the summer she was seven. With an
enviable bronze glow, she resembled an Indian of the Southwest. Half
her length was legs. "A dancer's legs," one of their friends commented,
and Isabel, her legs stretched out before her on the rug, smiled back
shyly, uncomprehending, with missing teeth. Caroline was grateful for
the missing teeth: they represented a visible lapse from perfection, even
if temporary. She didn't like the way the friend had looked at the child,
but told herself she was being absurd. Isabel was a baby. She liked to
wear her long hair severely tied behind with a ribbon. It swung over
her straight back like a skein of velvet. She winced and groaned every
morning under the hairbrush, while Caroline hardened her heart and
brushed on. "You can have it cut if you want." Isabel shook her head
with gentle stubbornness. "I like it long. Daddy likes it long." She was
strong, infatuated with life and her own beauty, spreading an entranc-
ing glow of goodwill. More than sheer infantile magic—she was truly
good, Caroline believed, the outer beauty an accurate portrait of the
inner. The fluctuations of emotion played openly on her face in
hundreds of tiny gradations in lips and eyes and color: reading her
expression, Caroline felt she saw through to the purity of nerve and
bone. In her seductive contradictions of innocence and subtlety she was
Ivan all over again, and she was bewitching.

They went, that summer, to an inn in the Berkshires for two weeks.
After a hike in the woods they lay on the large double bed, Isabel
resting between them, holding a hand on either side. Ivan was silent,

possibly dozing, while Isabel asked her usual questions and received the usual answers, from a script of unending fascination to her.

"So what do people do when they want to make a baby? Do they say, let's make a baby, just like that?"

"Well, not exactly. It happens in different ways. They usually both know if they want to."

"And then do they just go to bed and do it?"

"Yes."

"Do they have to take off all their clothes?"

"They don't have to, but they usually do."

"It must be so embarrassing. Do they have to be married?"

"No, they don't have to, but most people who have babies are. It's better for the baby that way."

The child suddenly clutched Ivan's arm. He started and blinked. "Let's get married!" she cried.

"What?"

"Let's get married."

"Oh. But I'm already married," he answered her, smiling. This, too, was from the script.

Instantly, with the fleetness of a butterfly, she was stretched out full length on top of him. "Well, let's make a baby anyway."

Ivan put his hands on her shoulders and laughed out loud. "I already made a baby."

"Isabel," said Caroline, "it's hot in here. Go and open the window, please."

Grunting with mild resentment, she climbed off Ivan and did as she was asked. "Anything to get me out of the way," she said good-naturedly.

Caroline blushed. "Come here," she said, smiling. She moved over to make room for Isabel on her right, away from Ivan, circling an arm around her and hugging her close. Her body was soft, immediately yielding. Despite herself, Caroline, too, yielded. "You know I don't want you out of the way." Isabel snuggled into her side. After a while Caroline added, "How did you get so clever?" But no one heard. They had both fallen asleep.

She watched them. They even slept alike, their brows slightly furrowed and their lips, the bowed, exquisitely articulated lips, barely parted. But Ivan, as usual, groped and clung; one leg was flung over her own, a heavy, comforting weight, his fist was pressed into the bend of her waist, and his chin had found her shoulder to lean on. Isabel's sleep was essentially solitary; Caroline might have been a wall or a pillow. She noted with a tinge of nostalgia how Isabel's primitive infant desires were restrained even in sleep: the renounced thumb came to rest gently on her lower lip, pulling it down to reveal the soft inner pink of her mouth.

The child had an unfair advantage, she thought. Isabel did things that she couldn't do. Evenings when she heard the click of the door— and she always heard it first—she raced through the living room to meet Ivan and leap up in his arms. When his hair periodically grew long enough Isabel would tie it back in a rubber band and bring him a mirror to see. He submitted like a ludicrous enchanted lover. Bottom and Titania, Caroline thought, looking on. After her bubble bath Isabel would run out, the huge flowered towel fastened like a sarong, and offer him her small shoulder to smell. Ivan rolled his eyes, sighed, and pretended to swoon.

oo oo oo
FANNY HOWE

Onset

As with a great storm or onset, she could hear through the walls of her body the hysteria of two whose voices hit a pitch neither male nor female. Getting fixed only took those noises and an interior silence, a moment which she knew every time. Age-old urge, emergency among the whirlpools, the fragments and sweeping curves of her torso. A sudden squall, the flutter of a breeze in her ear, and she was done.

She began to harden with the first one. A firm heel slid across the palm of her hand, under her navel, now like a moonsnail with a cat's eye at its apex. Her wastes, and its, moved in opposite directions from the nutrients. Her breasts tightened to tips of pain. She entered her psyche daily on rising, and like Clare who sucked the breast of Saint Francis, she frenziedly inhaled the Ave Maria. A he grew inside, or was a being. An expedition of several oar-ships.

Perfumes of the senses met a collection of bones and springs, and in her genitals a language of body fluids and secretions, tracts and tissues, bone marrow, breast milk, joint fluids—she had to think of these. The creation could only read itself!

She trudged up and down the island and daily visited beaches which were duneless but sided by slick streaks of beachgrass. The shadows of seagulls spilled along water's edges. Silk pennants fluttered over the breakwater and sometimes rain glistened in the dark. Fishing boats and cutters had black-green barnacled bottoms. The ruin of the deck and upper structures of many ships looked like fruit picked by sharks. Every stay and handrail held a bird in the dawn. Sticky oil, belched from a tunnel, had birds stuck on their pin-like toes. The poop went down, the bow went up, it was her body walking and a teeny skeleton inside like a cabin.

On the strand the waves were disorganized, they champed and struck each other, currents tugging at a mash of pebbles. Few shells, and those were cracked scallops or an old horseshoe crab. A flotsam of Styrofoam and plastic baggies. God's grave is blue and above. When you are living on the edge of your society are you closer to the center of the next era?

The embryo went to sleep early one night and in the liquidy darkness I stepped down the center of the road, by day bustling with cars and tourists. I walked toward the point which circled back along a harbor into town. I took a westerly direction knowing the sea would always have the last word.

This is the way to see a place—looking from darkness into lighted rooms. So the fetus derives nourishment from the light of oxygen. The white clapboard houses conformed like little tea kettles or mausoleums, with a staircase down the center, a kitchen beyond, and on either side a living room and study. The walls were marked with pictures of schooners and portraits of seafaring men. Streamlined launchers too, but no tramp steamers red with rust, no broad tugs, ropes or cables, or snakelike tubes winding from tanks; these were class ships. At twelve weeks the uterus is stretched like a canvas, larger than the pelvic cavity. It can be palpated above the symphysis pubis. But these rooms were white with polished wood. The furniture was stiff and economical. Like the ships themselves, they equated tidiness with worth. Old women dusted and drifted through the mannish spaces, giving to them the otherworldly sheen of sisters from the last century.

She was often sick, either hunched up or bent over, retching into a toilet bowl. Nature is extravagant. Her body was a difficulty in much the same spirit that a person's gender or income can be under certain conditions. Inside her eyes she saw placenta, membranes, amniotic fluids, cervical cul de sacs, a vulva and interior like the gums of an infant. However her mental dimensions tipped toward the metaphysical. G-d had been forced out of just such a world.

If there was such a quality as human nature, she now had to assume it was grounded in the machine she inhabited and which, again, inhabited her. The vagina and cervix in pregnancy are blue to purple. She was sure drug therapy was the best cure for depression. Motion was liberation from the gross inertia of the body which held swellings small as berries and full of air. You could be healed by leaping in the sea which is why she gravitated toward water towns. There flowering seaweed cooled her sore feet. The surface oysters with pearls embedded in pink flesh made her feel like a link of woman, coral to red, nameless as a breast. Now a hint of autumn let her spirits rise, her mind race.

I don't want to be a king or captain or bishop or chair. A summer of record-breaking heat and humidity created a swimming pollution, humans gasped like fish. In the seas a scandal of unsanitary objects. While five thousand small herrings nested in the stomach of a sperm whale and each one of them contained crabs who in turn had eaten algae, night storms kept the beaches lined with silver wiggling crill and human feces. The air stayed dense and dirty as if the rain itself had been a form of excretion. Birth is a calamity. So I cling to my infant and it to me.

I have become unified with my materials. Thorns made the beard of Jesus what it was. No field of blue flowers. No matter what I touch or work on, it's only me touching or working. Conversion is not putting on something new but shedding something old.

In her first pregnancy she found herself finally focussed on the presence of her body. Nothing was distracting from the fact that the mucus of the cervix is less viscid than sputum. She was conscious of how mechanistic and unnecessary a human life really was; every fact was an affirmation of perdition.

Rich and poor women look stark but strong. Clapboard houses, low to the ground, with protuberant fans and television antennae nestled in shrubbery lusciously green and dotted with flowers. Petunias, limp with purple trumpets too, proliferated. Some gardens had salmon-pink borders of impatiens and on the roadsides the clover was ripe, a farm was for sale, fresh baked pies were lined up on planks beside beach plum jelly and apple cinnamon. Mopeds and bikes cruised the narrow roads where she crawled. Pastures humped under her back in the long grass, the sky was often misty or gray. She wondered, when she woke out there one day, if the objects she saw on the left in her dreams were emanating from that side of her brain.

Well, I said, you sweep people away like a dream. I'm glad when you call to me, Let's go. Seeking face. I WILL seek your face.

Is it human nature to crave the love of indifferent people? Does a displaced center become a periphery? She certainly did, even while she sustained bonds to distant friends. Past their shoulders she always seemed to glimpse the image of someone who had forgotten she was alive and hardly cared to discover she was. One such person told her that the mirror for human nature was art and that the secret therefore of her essence could be found in the recognition she would feel before certain words and works. Without such recognition she could only feel revulsion toward the experience of producing more body fluids, another epiglottis, endometrium, and so on.

Pregnancy created a tie to her own accidental source. To view the condition as a disease which she had caught was to reject the knowledge of a human for its own nature. A plant might look like it's growing a beard but we know that it isn't.

She didn't remain as static as a plumed worm even—building its home in a papery tube.

She inhabited her inhabitant and kept on moving. The larvae of softshell clams do no less. In an environment that changes wildly, creation creates a lot of itself. In a fierce storm barnacles, worms and mussels reproduce in droves. If she wondered who really owned her hand, writing with a pen, and where she could be located, she now knew one thing at least and for the time being: she was present at her own life!

The collarlike erection on the beach was made by a moonsnail to protect her eggs. So she was an organism which existed alongside the other particulars in the universe. She was really here where the egg-cases of skates, called mermaid purses, are dry and black with two spiny tendrils at either end.

By accepting the fact of her existence she had to accept the terms in which science generally spoke of such facts. Herring gulls eat horseshoe crabs, but she turned away from the temptation of brutalism. She like some tried to believe that the secret name of the power that is the foreginning of everything was HUMAN. While the integrity of her pregnancy was maintained by high levels of estrogen and progesterone, her personal integrity was maintained by identifying with eremites.

She had begun to feel close to the ground. The poverty line was dollars above her, she who had been one of the working poor. America ran through her sleep too fast. But beach heather with its yellow spring blossoms was not her bed either. Grasshoppers belong to beach grass.

One morning a cloudbank slipped over the island like a smoker trailing around a garden. Seaweed in the cracks of rock and bits of sponge and seaside goldenrod held her lying in the sun. The trees were filmy, the national shades of noon still softened by immortal light. A caterpillar here, a snake there, by Labor Day most of the wildflowers were eliminated. Small baggy areas formed in the troughs between dunes, and she hid in them with a stolen apple pie. To be happy alone you don't need to be a martyr.

From some leaves thick as leather hung nuts, rocky brown ones with dimpled caps. Beach peas grew in the sand with wild cherry and beach plum. I'd eat kelp, sea lettuce, maybe even Irish moss. I didn't want to hitchhike at my age or in my condition but instead scuffed my sneakers through the sandy soil and twitched with the pains in my calves. Pork of veal, pork of veal, someone called in a room through the trees. The light seemed painted on the surface of each oak leaf. So I remembered artifice, I a free woman who had neither home nor office, and then I remembered d—th, and wept.

oo oo oo

MAXINE CHERNOFF

The Fetus _____

The fetus came up to me. It was a normal fetus—large, translucent head, stumpy arms and legs, a heart resembling a bird's nest visible through the chest cavity. It looked at me imploringly, pointing in its ambiguous way at something on my face. The fetus, it seemed, wanted to touch my glasses. I bent down slowly, so as not to startle it. It seemed to take hours and I realized how low I'd have to bend to accommodate my visitor. The touch of the fetus was the touch of someone groping to turn off an alarm. Inept and sleepy and furious all at once. In its small commotion the fetus knocked my glasses to the floor. I hesitated, not daring to speak, to see what it would do. The blurry fetus looked at me, turned and left abruptly as it had arrived. I wondered whether it wanted to wear my glasses for a moment or if its intention had been to touch my eye. When my daughter came home from school, I told her this story. Her eyes strained at mine; they had the same look I've detected when she's being lied to by a stranger.

oo oo oo

LAURA CHESTER

Who Knows _____

When I received Kate's note that said she was ten days late, I was also about seven days late, and thrilled, not so much for myself or for her, but for the amazing, unplanned synchronicity. I called her immediately to find out that Yes, she had taken the rabbit test. Positive.

"When the nurse announced the results, Mel yelled Great!"

"Great," I agreed.

"But no," she continued. "He thought I was positively *not* pregnant."

"Oh, I see. Not so great."

"Listen," Kate told me, "No one must know about this, not even Cynthia."

"How can we not tell Cynthia?"

"We just have to wait. I promised Mel I wouldn't tell anyone, because first of all, we're not quite sure, and I want him to feel like he can decide."

So Kate slipped off to have a secret lunch with her mother and spilled the baked beans, insisting that her mother tell no one, not even her father, and so meanwhile Kate's mother got desperate to relate the good news to someone, just to ease the burden of her happiness. What good is joy if you can't get rid of it a little!

I was very good and didn't let on, so that Kate could tell Cynthia herself, and then she told both of us that her mother now knew, but that Mel didn't know that her mother knew, and must not know, because the plan was, that she and Mel were going to tell Kate's parents together. Mel wanted to announce that he had decided to marry their daughter, and to give them a grandchild, all of which had to be received as Great News!

Although Cynthia now knows, we still can't tell Nancy, another best friend to all three of us. Even though I never did come right out and tell Nancy, when I said, "Poor Kate got sick last night at the concert," Nancy responded, "Well that's what happens when you're pregnant," and I went, "What?"

Nancy nodded slyly, "Listen girls. I've had an inkling of my own for a couple of weeks."

So we made Nancy promise not to tell anyone, especially not Kate. We didn't want our friend to mistrust us. So now Nancy knows, and Kate doesn't know, plus Kate's mother knows and Mel doesn't know, and neither does Kate's father.

But what if Nancy accidentally told Mel that Kate had told her mother, having to explain that it was just something a daughter couldn't keep back, but that he shouldn't let on that he knew that Kate's mother knew, so that Kate would finally be the only one who didn't know what.

ARLENE STONE

from: Son Sonnets _____

3

St. Valentine one month past prime when we
conceived you. My womb still jetted hearts
    in limpid
starts. Love, I was plunged like sparrow
by the earthward turbulent descent
of Cupid's icicle, liquescent arrow.
The roué held a rose between bicuspids.
His curls resembled chocolate swirls on candy.
Butts firm as nuts, as cherries ripe on flank
of rum, we lushed on Barricini satin.
Count moon times nine, pursuing arrow sky-
ward to find the baby centaur, a deep moon
    crescent
graven in his forehead where they pry
him from me; rope of honey. Proclaim two matins
before blood syrup bells upon my snowbank.

4

Once before there was *Selah*! such radiance.
I blew glass veins for you, three hundred sixty-
five, and drugged their vessels with fresh
    blood soup.
Your body cabinets I made two hundred
forty-eight; near twenty wings aswoop
to loop you prayershawl; rubies threw a pixie
light on six-pronged star of frankincense.
So guided were the stars to your menorah.
Nine candle branches had your tree, said those
who worshipped to the East, who brought for hair
a fine Nile cotton, and for skin, Egyptian
hemp. A crown of olive shone on two fair
married lions, upon a bed supposed
of velveteen, the night the sky was Torah.

oo oo oo

ALICIA OSTRIKER

Propaganda Poem: Maybe for Some Young Mamas _____

I. THE VISITING POET

(after reading the girls my old pregnancy poem
that I thought ripe and beautiful
after they made themselves clear it was ugly
after telling the girls I would as soon
go to my grave a virgin, god
forbid, as go to my grave without
ever bearing and rearing a child
I laughed
and if looks could kill I would
have been one dead duck in that
                so-called "feminist" classroom)

Oh young girls in a classroom
with your smooth skins like paper not yet written on
your good American bodies, your breasts, your bellies
fed healthy on hamburgers and milkshakes, almost
like photographs in solution half-developed
I leaned and strained toward you, trying to understand
what you were becoming
as you sat so quietly under the winter light
that fell into our classroom
and I tried, as a teacher, to transmit information
that's my job, knowledge like currency
you have to spend it

oh young mamas
no matter what your age is you
are born when you give birth
to a baby you start over

one animal

and both gently just slightly
separated from each other
swaying, swinging

25

like a vine, like an oriole nest
keep returning to each other
like a little tide, like a little wave
for a little while

        better than sex, that bitter honey, maybe
        could be the connection you've been waiting for
        because no man is god, no woman is a goddess
        we are all of us spoiled by that time

        but a baby
                any baby
                        your baby is
                                the
        most perfect human thing you can ever touch
        translucent
        and I want you to think about   touching
        and the pleasure of   touching
        and being touched by this most perfect thing
                this pear tree blossom
           this mouth these leafy hands these genitals
                like petals
           a warm scalp resting against your cheek
                fruit's warmth
                beginning—

Curtains curtains you say young girls
we want to live our lives
don't want the burden the responsibility
the disgusting mess
of children
we want our freedom and we want it now
I see you shudder truly and I wonder what
        kind of lives you want so badly
        to live or who has cut you with what axes
        from the sense of your
        flowing sap or why
        are you made of sand
young girls will you walk
out of this door and spend your substance freely
or who has shown to you the greedy mirror
the lying mirror
the desert
sand—

I am telling you and you can take me for a fool there is no
good time like the good time a whole mama
has with a whole little baby and that's
                                        where the first images
of deity came from—sister you know it's true
you know in secret how they
cut us down
                because who can bear the joy that hurts nobody
                the dazzling circuit of contact without dominance
                that by the way might make you less vulnerable
                to cancer and who knows what other diseases
                of the body
                because who can bear a thing that makes you happy
                and rolls the world a little way
                                        on forward
                                toward its destiny

                because a woman is acceptable if she is
                weak
                acceptable if she is a victim
                acceptable also if she is an angry victim ("shrew," "witch")
                a woman's sorrow is acceptable
                a deodorized sanitized sterilized antiperspirant
                grinning efficient woman is certainly acceptable

but who can tolerate the power of a woman
close to a child, riding our tides
into the sand dunes of the public spaces.

2. POSTSCRIPT TO PROPAGANDA

That they limit your liberty, of course,
entirely. That they limit your cash. That they limit your sleep.
Your sleep is a dirty torn cloth.
That they whine until you want to murder them. That their beauty
prevents you. That their eating and excreting exactly resembles
the slime-trails of slugs. On your knees you follow, cleaning,
unstaining. That they burn themselves, lacerate themselves, bruise
themselves. That they get ill. That you sit at their bedsides
exhausted, coughing, reading dully to them, wiping their foreheads
with wet washcloths to lower the fever, your life peeling away
from you like layers of cellophane. Of course.

That you are wheels to them. That you are grease.
An iron doorway they kick open, they run out, nobody has
remembered to close it. That their demanding is a grey north wind.
That their sullenness is a damp that rots your wood, their
malice a metal that draws your blood, their disobedience the fire that
burns your sacred book, their sorrows the webbing that entraps you
like a thrashing fish. That when your child grieves, mother,
you bend and grieve. That you disentwine yourself from them, lock
the pores of your love, set them at a distance. That in this
fashion the years pass, like calendar pages flipped in a silent
movie, and you are old, you are wrinkled as tortoises.

Come on, you daughters of bitches, do you want to live forever?

JAYNE ANNE PHILLIPS

Bluegill _____

Hello my little bluegill, little shark face. Fanged one, sucker, hermaphrodite. Rose, bloom in the fog of the body; see how the gulls arch over us, singing their raucous squalls. They bring you sweetmeats, tiny mice, spiders with clasped legs. In their old claws, claws of eons, reptilian sleep, they cradle shiny rocks and bits of glass. Boat in my blood, I dream you furred and sharp-toothed, loping in snow mist on a tundra far from the sea. I believe you are male; will I make you husband, uncle, brother? Feed you in dark movie houses of a city we haven't found? This village borders waves, roofs askew, boards vacant. I'll leave here with two suitcases and a music box, but what of you, little boot, little head with two eyes? I talk to you, bone of my coming, bone of an earnest receipt. I feel you now, steaming in the cave of the womb.

Here there are small fires. I bank a blaze in the iron stove and waken ringed in damp; how white air seeps inside the cracked houses, in the rattled doors and sills. We have arrived and settled in a house that groans, shifting its mildewed walls. The rains have come, rolling mud yards of fishermen's shacks down a dirt road to the curling surf. Crabs' claws bleach in spindled grass; dogs tear the discarded shells and drag them in rain. They fade from orange to peach to the pearl of the disembodied. Smells crouch and pull, moving in wet air. Each night crates of live crab are delivered to the smokehouse next door. They clack and crawl, a lumbering mass whose mute antennae click a filament of loss. Ocean is a ream of white meat, circles in a muscular brain. I eat these creatures; their flesh is sweet and flaky. They are voiceless, fluid in their watery dusk, trapped in nets a mile from the rocky cliffs. You are some kin to them, floating in your own dark sac.

Kelp floats a jungle by the pier, armless, legless, waving long sea hair, tresses submerged and rooty. These plants are bulbs and a nipple, rounded snouts weaving their tubular tails. Little boys find them washed up on the beach, wet, rubbery, smelling of salt. They hold the globular heads between their legs and ride them like stick horses. They gallop off, long tails dragging tapered in the sand. They run along the water in groups of three or four, young centaurs with no six-guns whose tracks evoke visions of mythical reptiles. They run all the way to the point, grow bored, fight, scatter; finally one comes back alone, preoccupied, dejected, dragging the desultory tail in one hand as the foamy surf tugs it seaward. I watch him; I pretend you see him too, see it all with your X-ray vision, your soft eyes, their honeycomb facets judging the souls of all failed boys. We watch the old ones, the young ones, the boats bobbing their rummy cargoes of traps and nets and hooks.

I sit at the corner table of the one restaurant, diner near the water where fishermen drink coffee at six A.M. I arrive later, when the place is nearly empty, when the sun slants on toward noon and the coffee has aged to a pungent syrup. The waitress is the postmaster's wife; she knows I get one envelope a month, that I cash one check at MacKinsie's Market, that I rent a postbox on a six-month basis. She spots my ringless hands, the gauntness in my face, the calcium pills I pull out of my purse in a green medicinal bottle. She recognizes my aversion to eggs; she knows that blur in my pupils, blur and flare, wavering as though I'm sucked inward by a small interior flame. You breathe, adhered to a cord. Translucent astronaut, your eyes change days like a calendar watch. The fog surrounds us, drifting between craggy hills like an insubstantial blimp, whale shape that breaks up and spreads. Rock islands rise from the olive sea; they've caught seed in the wind and sit impassive, totems bristling with pine. Before long they will split and speak, revealing a long-trapped Hamlin piper and a troop of children whose bodies are musical and perfect, whose thoughts have grown pure. The children translate each wash of light on the faces of their stone capsules; they feel each nuance of sun and hear the fog as a continuous sigh, drifted breath of the one giant to whom they address their prayers. They have grown no taller and experienced no disease; they sleep in shifts. The piper has made no sound since their arrival. His inert form has become luminous and faintly furred. He is a father fit for animalistic angels whose complex mathematical games evolve with the centuries, whose hands have become transparent from constant handling of quartz pebbles and clear agates. They have no interest in talk or travel; they have developed beyond the inhabitants of countries and communicate only with the unborn. They repudiate the music that tempted them and create it now within themselves, a silent version expressed in numerals, angles, complicated slitherings. They are mobile as lizards and opaque as those small blind fish found in the still waters of caves. Immortal, they become their own children. Their memories of a long-ago journey are layered as genetics: how the sky eclipsed, how the piped melody was transformed as they walked into the sea and were submerged. The girls and smaller boys remember their dresses blousing, swirling like anemones. The music entered a new dimension, felt inside them like cool fingers, formal as a harpsichord yet buoyant, wild; they were taken up with it days at a time. . . .

Here in the diner, there is a jukebox that turns up loud. High school kids move the tables back and dance on Friday nights. They are sixteen, tough little girls who disdain makeup and smoke Turkish cigarettes, or last year's senior boys who can't leave the village. Already they're hauling net on their fathers' boats, learning a language of profanity and back-slapping, beer, odd tumescent dawns as the other boats float out of sight. They want to marry at twenty, save money, acquire protection from the weather. But the girls are like colts, skittish and lean; they've read magazines, gone to rock concerts, experimented with drugs and each other. They play truant and drive around all day in VWs, listen to AM radio in the rain and swish of the wipers, dream of graduation and San Francisco, L.A., Mexico. They go barefoot in the dead of winter and seldom eat; their faces are pale and dewy from the moist air, the continuous rains. They show up sullen-eyed for the dances and get younger as the evening progresses, drinking grocery-store mixed drinks from thermoses in boys' cars. Now they are willing to dance close and imitate their mothers. Music beats in the floor like a heart; movie-theme certainty and the simple lyric of hold-me-tight. I pause on my nightly walks and watch their silhouettes on the windows; nearby the dock pylons stand up mossy and beaten, slap of the water intimate and old. Boys sit exchanging hopeful stories, smoking dope. Sometimes they whistle. They can't see my shape in my bulky coat. Once, one of them followed me home and waited beyond the concrete porch and the woodpile; I saw his face past the thrown ellipses of light. I imagined him in my bed, smooth-skinned and physically happy, no knowledge but intent. He would address you through my skin, nothing but question marks. Instructed to move slowly from behind, he would be careful, tentative, but forget at the end and push hard. There is no danger; you are floating, interior and protected; but it's that rhythmic lapsing of my love for you that would frighten; we have been alone so long. So I am true to you; I shut off the light and he goes away. In some manner, I am in your employ; I feed my body to feed you and buy my food with money sent me because of you. I am very nearly married to you; and it is only here, a northwestern fishing village in the rains, constant rain, that the money comes according to bargain, to an understanding conceived in your interest. I have followed you though you cannot speak, only fold, unfold. Blueprint, bone and toenail, sapphire. You must know it all from the beginning, never suffer the ignorance of boys with vestigial tails and imagined guns. I send you all these secrets in my blood; they wash through you like dialysis. You are the

animal and the saint, snow-blind, begun in blindness ... you must
break free of me like a weasel or a fox, fatherless, dark as the seals that
bark like haunted men from the rocks, far away, their calls magnified
in the distance, in the twilight.

Ghost, my solitaire, I'll say your father was a horse, a Percheron
whose rippled mane fell across my shoulders, whose tight hide glim-
mered, who shivered and made small winged insects rise into the air.
A creature large-eyed, velvet. Long bone of the face broad as a forearm,
back broad as sleep. Massive. Looking from the side of the face, a
peripheral vision innocent, instinctual.

But no, there were many fathers. There was a truck, a rattling of
nuts and bolts, a juggling of emergencies. Suede carpenter's apron spot-
ted with motor oil, clothes kept in stacked crates. There were hands
never quite clean and later, manicured hands. A long car with mechanical windows that *zimmed* as they moved smoothly up and down, im-
penetrable as those clear shells separating the self from a dreamed
desire (do you dream? of long foldings, channels, imageless dreams of
fish, long turnings, echoed sounds and shading waters). In between,
there were faces in many cars, road maps and laced boots, hand-printed
signs held by the highway exits, threats from ex-cons, cajoling sales-
men, circling patrolmen. There were counters, tables, eight-hour shifts,
grease-stained menus, prices marked over three times, regulars pathetic
and laughing, cheap regulation nylons, shoes with ridged soles, cream-
ers filled early as a truck arrives with sugared doughnuts smelling of
vats and heat. Men cursed in heavy accents, living in motor hum of the
big dishwashers, overflowed garbage pails, ouzo at the end of the day.
Then there were men across hallways, stair rails, men with offices,
married men and their secretaries, empty bud vase on a desk. Men in
elevators, white shirts ironed by a special Chinaman on Bleecker. San-
itary weekend joggers, movie reviewers, twenty-seventh floor, manufactured air, salon haircuts, long lunches, tablecloths and wine. Rooftop
view, jets to cut swelling white slashes in the sky. And down below,
below rooftops and clean charmed rhymes, the dark alleys meandered;
those same alleys that crisscross a confusion of small towns. Same
sideways routes and wishful arrivals, eye-level gravel, sooty perfumes,
pale grass seeding in the stones. Bronzed light in casts of season: steely
and blue, smoke taste of winters; the pinkish dark of any thaw; then
coral falling in greens, summer mix of rot and flowers; autumn a burnt
red, orange darkened to rust and scab. All of it men and faces, pro-
gression, hands come to this and you, grown inside me like one reminder.

He faced me over a café table, showed me the town on a map. No special reason, he said, he'd been here once; a quiet place, pretty, it would do. One geography was all he asked in the arrangement, the "interruption." He mentioned his obligation and its limits; he mentioned our separate paths. I don't ask here if they know him, I don't speculate. I've left him purely, as though you came to me after a voyage of years, as though you flew like a seed, saw them all and won me from them. I've lived with you all these months, grown cowish and full of you, yet I don't name you except by touch, curl, gesture. Wake and sleep, slim minnow, luminous frog. There are clues and riddles, pages in the book of the body, stones turned and turned. Each music lasts, forgetful, surfacing in the aisles of anonymous shops.

Music, addition and subtraction, Pavlovian reminder of scenes becoming, only dreamed. Evenings I listen to the radio and read fairy tales; those first lies, those promises. Directions are clear: crumbs in the woods, wolves in red hoods, the prince of temptation more believable as an enchanted toad. He is articulate and patient; there is the music of those years in the deep well, *plunk* of moisture, *whish* of the wayward rain, and finally the face of rescue peering over the stone rim like a moon. Omens burst into bloom; each life evolved to a single moment: the ugly natural, shrunken and wise, cradled in a palm fair as camellias.

Knot of cells, where is your voice? Here there are no books of instructions. There is the planed edge of the oaken table, the blond rivulets of the wood. There is a lamp in a dirty shade and the crouched stove hunkering its blackness around a fiery warmth. All night I sit, feeling the glow from a couch pulled close to the heat. Stirring the ashes, feeding, feeding, eating the fire with my skin. The foghorn cries through the mist in the bay: *bawaah, bawaah*, weeping of an idiot sheep, steady, measured as love. At dawn I'm standing by the window and the fishing boats bob like toys across the water, swaying their toothpick masts. Perfect mirage, they glisten and fade. Morning is two hours of sun as the season turns, a dime gone silver and thin. The gnarled plants are wild in their pots, spindly and bent. Gnats sleep on the leaves, inaugurating flight from a pearly slime on the windowpane. Their waftings are broken and dreamy, looping in the cold air of the house slowly, so slowly that I clap my hands and end them. Staccato, flash: that quick chord of once-upon-a-time.

Faraway I was a child, resolute, small, these same eyes in my head sinking back by night. Always I waited for you, marauder, collector, invisible pea in the body. I called you stones hidden in corners, paper fish with secret meanings, clothespin doll. Alone in my high bed, the dark, the dark; I shook my head faster, faster, rope of long hair flying across my shoulders like a switch, a scented tail. Under the bed, beyond the frothy curtain duster, I kept a menagerie of treasures and dust: discarded metallic jewelry, glass rhinestones pried from their settings, old gabardine suitcoat from a box in the basement, lipsticks, compacts with cloudy mirrors, slippers with pompoms, a man's blue silk tie embossed with tiny golf clubs. At night I crawled under wrapped in my sheets, breathing the buried smell, rattling the bed slats with my knees. I held my breath till the whole floor moved, plethora of red slashes; saw you in guises of lightning and the captive atmosphere.

Now a storm rolls the house in its paws. Again, men are lost and a hull washes up on the rocks. All day search copters hover and sweep. Dipping low, they chop the air for survivors and flee at dusk. The bay lies capped and draggled, rolling like water sloshed in a bowl. Toward nightfall, wind taps like briers on the windowpanes. We go out, down to the rocks and the shore. The forgotten hull lies breaking and splintered, only a slab of wood. The bay moves near it like a sleeper under sheets, murmuring, calling more rain. Animal in me, fish in a swim, I tell you *everything drowns*. I say *believe me if you are mine*, but you push like a fist with limbs. I feel your eyes searching, your gaze trapped in the dark like a beam of light. Then your vision transcends my skin: finally, I see them too, the lost fishermen, their faces framed in swirling hair like the heads of women. They are pale and blue, glowing, breathing with a pulse in their throats. They rise streaming tattered shirts, shining like mother-of-pearl. They rise moving toward us, roundmouthed, answering, answering the spheres of your talk. I am only witness to a language. The air is yours; it is water circling in like departure.

FULL FLOWER

oo oo oo

ELIZABETH HAY

from: The Snow was Burning _____

One summer it got so hot that everyone forgot their names. They couldn't remember who they were. For a time they looked for their lost names but after a while they forgot to do even that. They just sat still.

One person had a rocking chair. She rocked until she fell asleep. In her dream Canada and cool made the same sound.

Each person in turn sat in the rocking chair, each person dreamed a name, and on waking told what it was. All the names were variations of cool. Siberia Cool, Pelly Cool, Inuvik Cool, etc. In this way they were all named again.

One woman wanted a name for her newborn child. She thought of Snow. North. Marten. Loon. She got out an atlas and it fell open not at a map but at a section called Polar Regions, under the larger heading of The Diversity of Life. She read that tundra is land from which the ice retreated 8000 years ago. Tundra remembers the ice: it has only a thin covering of soil. She thought of the face of a burn victim. It remembers the fire.

That summer everything broke except the heat. Dishes, cars, machines. But the heat went on and on.

People started to think about how to break the heat. One person went looking for a hairline crack in the heat. She went out onto a lake and the air was like a porcelain glaze two inches from her eyes. She paddled away from the air but it followed her. She was the vase, she realized. The hairline crack was in her!

So then she examined herself and found a faint line running down her belly. She hit the line with all her strength and out popped a baby. Immediately she felt cool.

She started breaking more things. Soon everything was broken and the world was much cooler.

oo oo oo

ANNE TYLER

from: *Breathing Lessons* _____

If Fiona remarried she would most likely acquire a new mother-in-law. Maggie hadn't considered that. She wondered if Fiona and this woman would be close. Would they spend their every free moment together, as cozy as two girlfriends?

"And suppose she has another baby!" Maggie said.

Ira broke off his boom-das to ask, "Huh?"

"I saw her through that whole nine months! What will she do without me?"

"Who're you talking about?"

"Fiona, of course. Who do you think?"

"Well, I'm sure she'll manage somehow," Ira said.

Maggie said, "Maybe, and maybe not." She turned away from him to look out at the fields again. They seemed unnaturally textureless. "I drove her to her childbirth classes," she said. "I drilled her in her exercises. I was her official labor coach."

"So now she knows all about it," Ira said.

"But it's something you have to repeat with each pregnancy," Maggie told him. "You have to keep at it."

She thought of how she had kept at Fiona, whom pregnancy had turned lackadaisical and vague, so that if it hadn't been for Maggie she'd have spent her entire third trimester on the couch in front of the TV. Maggie would clap her hands briskly—"Okay!"—and snap off the *Love Boat* rerun and fling open the curtains, letting sunshine flood the dim air of the living room and the turmoil of rock magazines and Fresca bottles. "Time for your pelvic squats!" she would cry, and Fiona would shrink and raise one arm to shield her eyes from the light.

"Pelvic squats, good grief," she would say. "Abdominal humps. It all sounds so gross." But she would heave to her feet, sighing. Even in pregnancy, her body was a teenager's—slender and almost rubbery, reminding Maggie of those scantily clad girls she'd glimpsed on beaches who seemed to belong to a completely different species from her own. The mound of the baby was a separate burden, a kind of package jutting out in front of her. "Breathing lessons—really," she said, dropping to the floor with a thud. "Don't they reckon I must know how to breathe by now?"

"Oh, honey, you're just lucky they offer such things," Maggie told her. "*My* first pregnancy, there wasn't a course to be found, and I was scared to death. I'd have loved to take lessons! And afterward: I remember leaving the hospital with Jesse and thinking, 'Wait. Are they going to let me just walk off with him? I don't know beans about babies! I don't have a license to do this. Ira and I are just amateurs.' I mean you're given all these lessons for the unimportant things—piano-playing, typing. You're given years and years of lessons in how to balance equations, which Lord knows you will never have to do in normal life. But how about parenthood? Or marriage, either, come to think of it. Before you can drive a car you need a state-approved course of instruction, but driving a car is nothing, nothing, compared to living day in and day out with a husband and raising up a new human being."

Which had not been the most reassuring notion, perhaps; for Fiona had said, "Jiminy," and dropped her head in her hands.

"Though I'm certain you'll do fine," Maggie said in a hurry, "And of course you have me here to help you."

"Oh, jiminy," Fiona said.

Ira turned down a little side road called Elm Lane—a double string of tacky one-story cottages with RVs in most of the driveways and sometimes a sloping tin trailer out back. Maggie asked him, "Who will wake up in the night now and bring her the baby to nurse?"

"Her husband, one would hope," Ira said. "Or maybe she'll keep the baby in *her* room this time, the way you should have had her do last time." Then he gave his shoulders a slight shake, as if ridding himself of something, and said, "What baby? Fiona's not having a baby; she's just getting married, or so you claim. Let's put first things first here."

Well, but first things weren't put first the time before; Fiona had been two months pregnant when she married Jesse. Not that Maggie wanted to remind him of that. Besides, her thoughts were on something else now. She was caught by an unexpected, piercingly physical memory of bringing the infant Leroy in to Fiona for her 2 a.m. feeding— that downy soft head wavering on Maggie's shoulder, that birdlike mouth searching the bend of Maggie's neck inside her bathrobe collar, and then the close, sleep-smelling warmth of Jesse's and Fiona's bedroom. "Oh," she said without meaning to, and then, "Oh!" For there in Mrs. Stuckey's yard (hard-packed earth, not really a yard at all) stood a wiry little girl with white-blond hair that stopped short squarely at her jawline. She had just let go of a yellow Frisbee, which sailed shuddering toward their car and landed with a thump on the hood as Ira swung into the driveway.

oo oo oo

SUMMER BRENNER

Blissed Raga _____

I

Before you were born darling
I carried you on my lap the prince
    of whales and I huffed and I puffed
through the great acline making our own
    mountain from testaments of wet love
Love's labor to skin to blood
    to cellular surprise

We got to be the miracle of Life
We got to be Life Making

got to got to got to got to
yes you got to

II

I wrote 9 month songs
of the newborn of the birth
For the orifice
    hangars of passage
and pursuit of light

For the infants of Tibet
    whose tall fathers hold them
higher even higher
whenever the sun can come through
the clouds of the Himalayas
Their fathers hold them up
    that they might know the sun

I opened my legs in Santa Cruz
that you would know the sun
    and seek it
And shoot out
blue as an iris
wet as a whale

wet as a whistle
hungry and afraid for the breast
   of an unknown mother
the heart of a long gone pa

III

Songs of the nines
Amelie singing her own
Back 30 years ago
Remember
We were dancing on the Cosmic Sea
Everyone was there
There that place
where it is all so with all
We fuck for it

IV

And later
after you were born
dear Felix
a woman spotting your naked bottom
how did she put it she said
Honey you sure were making love
Honey that baby is what I call making love
Honey got to got to got to got to

ISABEL HUGGAN

The Violation _____

It had been one of those January whiteouts, the kind of storm that obliterates landscape and leaves you with no sense of place. When we looked out at the dawn the wind had died and the snow was smooth as far as we could see, marred only by the tops of fence posts sticking out like cigarette butts down the lane. Ray said right away that he'd just snowshoe out to the main road and hitch a lift into town, and would I call the vice principal at eight and arrange for someone to take his first period French in case he was late. And would I also call Garnet to come 'round and do the lane since it looked as if the worst was over.

Once Ray was out the door I made the calls and settled into the wood stove warmth of the kitchen, comfortable in the padded rocker by the window. I was five months pregnant, barely showing, but conscious of every kick and flutter inside my rounding belly. It was all happening so slowly, far too slowly. I felt dragged down, as if the new weight in my body were pulling me under. Some days I felt I could hardly move, and spent hour after hour wrapped in a shawl, dreaming and discontent. I like changes to be immediate and definite, and it seemed then as if all the changes in my life were subtle and organic.

Oh, the move from the city had been definite enough, and I had relished that, had known exactly where and what I was. But since July, when we'd taken over this old farm in the Valley, I had felt myself slipping and spinning, the nausea of those first few months of pregnancy like motion sickness. Dizzy and disoriented, I could simply not believe that this was the beginning of putting down roots. I longed for time to collapse, so that we would not have to endure the process, could instead suddenly be what we wished to become—real, country people, whose lives would be one with the land.

We knew that up and down the concession there was talk about how long we'd last, and probably the placing of small bets as to the actual date we'd give up and vacate, hightail it back to some highrise. We had doubts too, but we'd persevered through a difficult fall and had gained confidence from that. I felt good thinking of all the work we'd already accomplished, the new skills we were acquiring. We were trying to become as self-sufficient as possible—but, of course, there were all kinds of problems. Like the lane. We couldn't manage it ourselves, so we did what most of our neighbors did and called Garnet, who'd dig you out for a price. He was the kind of crafty farmer who survived best in the Valley; who could profit even from bad weather.

Garnet had cleared us out to the road five times so far that winter, and twice he'd come in for coffee when his rounds had brought him to our house after supper. Ray and I had been eagerly hospitable, anxious to make a good impression on someone who obviously carried gossip from kitchen to kitchen. I served fruitcake and refrained from comment on his rural and right-wing opinions about the unemployed, Quebec, the Milk Board and the high cost of education. Partly I was being polite and politic, taking on what I believed to be the expected role of a farm wife. But partly my silence was because Garnet was like a magnet, gathering up all my particles of dissent and leaving me empty-handed, mesmerized by his down-home logic. And by his eyes.

Garnet was well into his fifties, a squat man whose large head sat squarely on broad shoulders, whose feet planted themselves as if each step meant business. His solid body and coarse features were a startling contrast to large soft brown eyes, the kind of eyes you would call sexy in another kind of face.

The noise of the plough woke me from my dozing in the chair after lunch, and I looked out to see Garnet's pumpkin-coloured rig pitting itself against the heavy drifts. Something dinosaur-like about the machine gave the scene an animal dimension so that Garnet seemed like a prehistoric cowboy, riding against the herds of snow. As if he had caught my thoughts, at that moment he looked toward the house and waved his cap in the air above his head. An old bronco buster at the edge of the ice age.

I moved away from the window then, over to the stove where what was left of the chicken soup I'd had for lunch sat cooling. I poured it into an enamel dish and was fastening on a wax paper cover when Garnet knocked at the door. I could see him through the frosted glass, standing on the porch, his breath rising in clouds around him. I unlatched the door and he stepped on to the rope mat inside.

"Hi," I said. "Trouble?"

"Nope, just thought I'd leave her sit for a minute, she's been going full tilt all morning. Thought I could warm up too, and ask for a cup of coffee," he said, pulling the door shut behind him. "Saw you there at the window, figured you weren't too busy to give a fellow some."

"Well, sure," I said, a little taken aback by his assumption. He was right, of course, I hadn't been doing anything. I'd only been sitting there, staring out at all that white. But still, his attitude bothered me. "Cream and sugar, isn't it?"

"Yup," he said. "And say, look now, would you make me a sandwich to go with that? I don't know when I'm going to finish doing all the lanes on the route today, the way this snow has packed in. I could be real late getting home."

That said he removed his cap, parka and boots, then began to strip off the heavy overalls he wore on top of his everyday clothes. I stood by the sink, immobile, but moved inwardly by a flood of feelings I find difficult to name even now. Part of my nature responded with pride that one of the locals would choose my kitchen for his lunch, sure that he'd get a good bite to eat. The image of myself as bountiful earth mother rose up glimmering in the winter sunlight.

But there was something else, a kind of instinctive suspicion. A quivering in the air. I was a doe in the forest, nostrils dilated to sniff the wind, catching the scent of the hunter. All my womanly conditioning to set forth food to fill men's bellies was being thwarted by another more powerful urge that said run, hide, take cover. This is male, this is dangerous. The terror was a mindless thing, starting at the base of my abdomen and spreading up and out my limbs, as if my body knew more than my brain could admit.

It was the way he took off his clothes. So casual, so cocksure, confidently taking over my kitchen. His eyes glowed in his ruddy face, and he smiled expectantly, waiting for me to move, to walk across the scrubbed pine floor to the breadbox, to begin waiting on him. My mother harped at us all for years: "I've waited on you hand and foot, and what thanks do I get? You've treated me like dirt, the lot of you." Never that role for me, I vowed.

But no sooner had my heart welled up in indignation, than embarrassment made me recoil. In the breadbox, only stale, store-bought bread. Humiliation above all others, to be caught short. And I was caught by the pull of wanting to please, to serve, and pushed by the wordless voices in my blood, warning me of danger.

I looked over my shoulder at Garnet, who sat there in that stolid, silent way of farmers, waiting. I was about to offer him the leftover chicken soup instead, when the voice found words.

Warning me: You know, if you go to a lot of trouble and fuss over this lunch, Garnet's going to get the idea you like him dropping in like this. He'll think you're lonely and he'll make a point of stopping by every time he's out. Why, look at him, even today, he's watching every move you make with those big brown eyes of his, and don't think for a moment he's not having ideas. He's just waiting to see how interested you are.

And the voices led me to a courtroom, where I shrank before the defense lawyer's cross-examination.

"So you *say* he forced his attentions upon you. But haven't you already admitted that you made it abundantly clear to the accused that he was welcome? In fact, *more* than welcome? Did you not offer him homemade chicken soup? And grilled cheese sandwiches with chili sauce on the side?"

The knowing leer, playing now to the jury. "I ask you! Would a woman trying to discourage a man's attentions serve him a lunch like that? Everyone knows the adage that the way to a man's heart is through his stomach. Is it any wonder then that this normal man, with normal male appetites, thought he was being offered a little more than lunch?" Another leer.

And I see myself dissolving in tears, accused of seducing poor Garnet with my country cooking.

No, I decided, I'll not take the chance of serving him soup, stale bread is all the old bugger will get from me.

Unnerved by the clarity of my imagination, I let the bread knife slip from my hand and it clattered to the floor, taking with it a dollop of the sandwich spread I was slathering on the dry bread. I bent down to retrieve the knife, and as I was wiping the pale glop off the floor, looked over at Garnet. He was sitting sideways on his chair, smiling cheerfully at my clumsiness, as if I had done it to amuse him. He had finished rolling three cigarettes, and had begun to smoke one.

"Listen," I said, in my most apologetic tone, "this isn't going to be much of a lunch, I'm afraid. With the storm and all we haven't got a lot on hand. We're out of milk, do you mind if I use powdered for your coffee?" With that, I plopped in a spoonful of instant milk powder, turning the instant coffee a sickening grey brown, with little lumpy white bits floating on the top. I set the cup and the plate in front of Garnet, and sat down at the table across from him. I noticed then that he'd been tapping the ashes from his cigarette into his leathery hand, and I got up and brought him an ashtray from the cupboard. I felt his eyes upon me as I moved.

When he reached out for the ashtray he seemed to contrive to touch my hand, I was sure of it, and I flinched at that contact like someone burned. My face felt as if there were small flames licking around my cheekbones. Ignited by fear, by the knowledge that he could reach out and with one swat of his enormous flat hands draw me up against the tobaccoey stench of his red and black plaid shirt. And in this place, in this snowbound and desolate valley, what could I do?

There was the irony. Back in the crime-rampant city I had been safer than here. At least there I was so used to being afraid I would never have let a man in the apartment while Ray was out, let alone serve him lunch. Safety in numbers, safety in cynicism, no good to me now.

I looked over at Garnet and could see by the way he set his teeth into the second bite of his sandwich that it was just as awful as I thought. But he kept his country courtesy intact and munched the horrible thing slowly and carefully, as if he were savouring it. He took my sitting down again as a signal to talk, and started, as one might expect, with the weather. This led him to a theme for which I felt some sympathy, that people today expect life to be easy and aren't prepared to cope with hardships. Worse than that, he went on, they have a diminishing sense of foresight.

"Just no common sense at all," Garnet said, stopping to take a small sip at his coffee. "Take that new young couple on the fifth, they build a house and they build it facing square northwest. So what do they have this winter? They've got drifts half covering their front picture window and a heat bill that's sky high. If they'd taken the time to ask a few people around here, they'd have that bungalow as cozy and snug . . ." He stopped, this time to finish the last bite of the sandwich; I rose, to indicate I could make him another, but hoping in my heart he would take it as a signal that lunch was over.

"Now you and Ray, for example," he said then, his broad face spread further by a smile. "You seem to be doing fine your first winter up here, but I'll bet you still have a lot to learn from us old-timers. Yup, some of us old dogs know a few more tricks than the young pups do, if you know what I mean." And he winked, and smiled.

I was filled with an unclean horror, a knowledge I didn't want, the way I feel when someone tells a dirty joke and says "Get it?" and I get it and wish with all my heart I didn't. An old dog, yes, of course that's what Garnet was. Under those few layers of clothes he was as much an animal as any rutting ram or bull or stallion, the same male energy runs them all.

I stood by the counter and took the knife in my hand, and gestured toward the loaf of bread, but Garnet shook his head. "I suppose that's true, we have a lot to learn," I said, thinking maybe not the knife, maybe the scalding kettle. No, that might burn me as well. And I saw myself suddenly standing over the prone body of poor Garnet, the knife in my hand, dripping his blood. Having killed, to save myself from what? A few searching kisses from a man testing out his age? A pat or two, a nuzzle, a little warmth and touching of youth? Would I really stab living flesh to protect myself from so little?

Not for myself, I thought, but for the baby. To save that small curled-up being from harm I would do anything.

Again, the voices echo in a courtroom, and again I am in the witness box, head lowered. Another defense lawyer, this time my own. "You see before you the victim of hormonal derangement, the temporary madness of the prepartum female, her enticement of the victim followed by her predictable revulsion with the incident, ending in violence and blood shed in self-defense. Have pity in your hearts, ladies and gentlemen of the jury . . ."

"Sorry," I said, "pardon?"

"I said, you don't have any family do you?" Garnet was leaning forward, he had a sly look around the eyes.

Oh god, I thought, he's checking to see there's no one in the house with me, he wants to make sure he has me all alone. I must act as if I'm not aware. As if everything were normal.

"Well, not yet," I replied, smoothing my loose-fitting shirt over my stomach, "but we will, come the spring." I smiled significantly, and at the moment was filled with a tremendous surge of power, as if, miraculously, there were adrenalin flowing from my womb.

"For the luvva mike," said Garnet, sitting back in his chair. "That's a real surprise, that is!"

"We're just starting to tell people," I began to explain. "But we haven't told any of the neighbours yet. The only person around here who knows is Joe Warrington. He sold Ray some nice white pine for the cradle he's making. And oh, his wife, she knows, she's teaching me how to knit and crochet so I can make my own things for the baby."

I was on safe ground now, inside the holy porch of motherhood. The menace in the air evaporated like mist in sunlight. The fetus kicked inside me. I was sacred, a repository for another human being, no longer a sexual object. He would not touch me now, I was sure. A farmer would have too much respect for these forces of life. I could no longer be harmed.

Garnet's face clouded as I kept talking about the plans we had for making the front room a nursery, and how glad we were we'd be raising our children in the country, not the city. As I chattered happily he gathered up his tobacco pouch and his yellow packet of papers, put them in his breast pocket and stood up. I was so startled by his sudden rising that I involuntarily gasped, and my hands flew to my chest like those of a timid maiden aunt. He looked at me, his liquid eyes full and deep.

"Can't be sitting here all day, there's work to do out there," he said, and reached for his heavy overalls. He drew them on, and then his parka, and sat down again to pull on his flapping-tongued boots. The room was silent except for the sound of laces through leather and the shift of logs in the stove. Embarrassed, I felt I should move toward him in some way, to find out why he was leaving so abruptly. Had I been wrong all along? Was he shy of baby talk the way some men are? Or had he really hoped to seduce me, and was his ardour cooled by the notion of my occupied belly?

"Do you have a family?" I asked. It seemed, once spoken, too personal a question.

"Well, now, I'll tell you," he said, arranging his cap on his head. "I didn't want to say this but on second thought I will. The wife and I don't have children, and not because we intended it that way. Oh, we're used to it now okay, but we started out all fired up like you, and it took us a long while to get used to life the way it had to be. She had two miscarriages to begin, and then a stillborn boy and then more trouble after that, so the doctor told us to put a stop to trying. And I'm not complaining, you understand, it's just the way things are."

I felt tears prickling the corners of my eyes, and a warm saltiness at the back of my throat. But Garnet had an air of composure, as he leaned on the back of his chair and spoke in that direct, hypnotic way.

"And I guess I should say what I think, which is don't go getting yourself all tied up in this here coming baby. Because it might work out and it might not. And if it doesn't, there has to be more to your life than all these plans. Don't plan too much on anything. You never know from one season to the next. You'll find that out, farming."

He put on his fur-lined mitts and opened the door.

"I didn't mean to come over all gloomy," he said, "so that's why I thought I better get on my way. Thanks for the lunch, it was just fine." He stepped out into the bright winter light, smiling.

"Thank you," I said, not knowing what I was thanking him for. I didn't feel grateful. I felt wounded and angry. He had violated me with that sad story as surely as if he had raped me. Like a wicked angel he had brought a message of destruction and despair. What right had he to barge in here and tell me what to hope or not to hope?

Garnet boarded his machine, and I closed the door after him, leaning against it. I felt stricken and cheapened by my stupid fears and caught now in a trap of superstition and uncertainty. I put my hands on my bulging abdomen, feeling for a sudden reassuring jut of life. Nothing. Nothing. Was Garnet some prophet sent to forewarn me of disaster?

What could I be certain of, after all? Outside, the snow stretched flawlessly across the fields, blotting out all the familiar marks and meanings. And here, inside, there were no signposts for the journey either.

oo oo oo

LAURA CHESTER

Suckle Sex _____

Huge hungry horse lips close over my breast and pull. I watch in astonishment— How does it know not to eat me up? Then Luna the cat climbs to feed. Her lily-spike incisors could puncture, her kneading feet could claw, but it doesn't hurt— She is teaching me how and what I will do. Relax. Give in. Give way to the temple on the tit, the little hut of flesh that stands and sings for the letting down of milk. A system of blue-veined rivers runs uphill, to this well, to this sort of source. How nice to let the body offer on its own, first comfort. My animal man and I are learning a new way, concave convex, pregnant as sensuously full. My breasts before lay dormant, occasionally cozy as sand dune, but now irrigation makes good the soil, firms up my juicy hillocks, which want soft squeeze and so much attention, so much more a part of the full bodily tension to peak and release in swells. A part of the wave hard hump tidal zing that floats the body to a tumble. The rumble and subsiding. Then again—waters run inland run wild through fern shelter and low hanging coils, a jungle for the wet mouth that twirls out of line into circles, that goes for the neck meat, the lover's tunnel, his prick full-fleshed and blood-long, into my mouth, me squirming delightful. I want him to come in, come on in and be welcome. His weight— Want his body, I want to be ground with that circular motion, the grip rock and holding, want to live out the dream of the cat heat, how she raises her raw butt for relief for the come on, and enter mine too, backdoors, my ass in the air, my claws in the feather pillow, for the carving of the groove, the smooth sink, the pink meat pounding, till all is contentment. When I say I am feeling more mammal, I don't mean a cow to responses, but a milked and contented cow-feel might not be a bad one to have now and again. Contentment of every cell I say, as mud is relaxed, and the slow awakening when nothing calls— Then sun snuggles up and around you. And the dream is persuaded to surface, like the enormous one-layer cake that rose up in the backseat, suspended in a liquid like jello. We bite right into the energy cookie, that first cake, placenta, our round and tummy baked creation. All enjoy their joy one way or another— Frog thumbs in armpits, cat teeth in cat neck, plunging in for both to swim in whatever way they ever imagined.

oo oo oo

MIRIAM SAGAN

Armed Robbery _____

The day I held up the 7-Eleven I was in a bad mood. I had morning sickness until late afternoon and there was nothing to eat in the house. The heat of late June lay over the bad end of town. I lay on the couch reading *From Russia With Love* and drinking flat ginger ale without ice. Then I took the gun out of the shoebox where it sat on top of a pair of red Italian sandals with dirty heels. I took the gun, got into the truck, drove down Agua Fria, and parked outside the 7-Eleven. I could have simply taken a twenty out of my underwear drawer but I was in no mood to go shopping. I walked into the 7-Eleven tripping over my flip flops. My armpits smelled of dust. Inside I put the gun on the counter. "This is a hold-up," I said to the lady behind the counter. She was a Spanish lady of about fifty. Her name tag read: Maureen. "What's your problem?" said Maureen. "I'm going to have a baby," I said peevishly. "Does that give you the right to come busting in here?" she said. "I'm a wreck," I said. "I should have gotten my Ph.D. in English literature like my mother wanted me to." "Shit," said Maureen. "You think you're the first woman in the world to have a baby? Calm down girl. You'll feel a lot better when you get into the second trimester. Right now your hormones are just going wild." "And I'm sick to my stomach all the time." "Crackers," said Maureen. "You need crackers." She pulled down a box of saltines for me. Then she opened a can of Diet Pepsi for herself and poured me a glass of apple juice. "I can't pay for this you know," I said. "That's alright," said Maureen. "Consider it part of the hold-up."

MIRIAM SAGAN

Heroines _____

Grace is four months pregnant. She lives on her ranch up near El Rito. In January she will have to drive the gorge at night over sleet to get to the birth center. When will she be able to walk to the farthest ridge again? She thinks she could still do it, but it would take all day now, and she would have to carry water. It isn't worth it. Grace has an amniocentesis in Los Alamos and a midwife in Taos. As a maternity outfit she is wearing a lot of red lipstick. Her child will be born under the sign of Capricorn. She will have to use Pampers because the nearest laundromat is in Espanola. Grace has gained twenty pounds from eating cake.

Mary Ann will have her baby at home in three weeks. It is a good way to frighten her mother-in-law. Mary Ann is an ex-heroin addict which now makes her very suburban. She despises Pampers and will use the diaper service and bio-bottoms. Mary Ann will not have the baby innoculated because she has developed a phobia about needles. She refuses all tests because she is only thirty, has one healthy child already, and would never consider an abortion. Her child will be born under the sign of Libra. She is wearing a purple mumu and a migraine headache. Mary Ann has gained sixty-five pounds and her husband won't let her cut her hair.

Miriam is afraid of her doctors although their first names are Beatrice, Laura, and Maria—three important ladies of the Middle Ages— Dante's muse, Petrarch's muse, and the Virgin Mother of God. Miriam's husband has tested negative for Tay-Sachs. She is relieved, but fears he may not really be Jewish. Her child will be born under the sign of Aquarius. She wears a Japanese maternity skirt where the elastic goes under the belly. She has lost eleven pounds from morning sickness that went on all day. Prenatal vitamins make her gag.

Mary Ann knows that her husband will get stoned again when she is in the middle of labor. She does not mind though because she loves him, and because he once said: Like wow, being pregnant is like surfing, sometimes you get a good wave, sometimes a bummer. He has seen her with her legs spread and with a needle in her arm. Miriam worries that her husband is not as pregnant as she is, perhaps he is getting off too lightly. He will believe it all much more when he sees the baby. For the moment, he likes it that her breasts are getting bigger. Miriam is thinking she might be an unwed teenage mother walking along upper Broadway and so she is grateful to be married in Santa

Fe. Mary Ann is thinking about green beans, her Texas grandmother, and the way morphine feels about four seconds after it enters your vein. Grace is wondering how she will ever ride her mare again. She is thinking about blue horses seen from a distance, in the far field, against a rose-colored butte. She is thinking about a far blue field.

oo oo oo

JOAN SLESINGER LOGGHE

Madonna of the Peaches ─────────────

I said,
take my belly
in the peaches.

We stood amid bees
before the blossoms blew
turned brown, then into fruit.

And I was all belly
turned this way
and that in the leaves.

Photos so young and taut
smooth surface like a globe
like a pink balloon before the party.

Like Venus of Laussel
on Kodak paper. My moment
amid the spring buzzing.

I said, leave out my face
with its traces of worry
and gray hair.

But my hand on my belly,
my left hand older than peach trees,
my workaday hand.

Those veins give shadow
to a presence, ancient
closer to the Goddess.

EDNA O'BRIEN

from: *The Country Girls Trilogy* _____

"There's a real live problem facing us, get your thinking cap on," I told her.

"What?" said she.

"The old, old story," I said, sort of singing it, to make it less awful.

"Love," she said. If you say potato famine she'll say love.

"Preg," I said, remembering that I'd said it to her before when we were in Dublin and she'd said, "How?" and I'd said, "The usual way," and she'd said something else, and I'd said it was easier than owning two coats. Well, the conversation repeated itself, verbatim. At least this time we had money and we had drink, and she didn't know it, but I had a gallon tin of castor oil in the shed, if the worse really came to the worst.

"But children are nice," she said. "You're fond of Cash."

"It helps," I said, because she may have got a scholarship but in some ways she's a moron, "if they have a trace of their father's eyes, ears, nose, feet, or something. Would I be that frantic if it was ortho-dox?"

It dawned on her. She wanted to know who. What was he like? What was it like? Did I see him often? Was I in love? Should we go and see him? See him! He'd bolted to Greece! I was in two minds whether I should tell her or not that it was all her fault. But the thought of a big ream of apology stopped me. It was action we needed.

You won't believe it but she asked me was I hoping it would be a boy or a girl.

"Twins," I said. "Two of each."

She got all soppy then about irony, telling me a card she'd seen in a For Sale window which said UNWORN MATERNITY DRESS, FINE GRAY CHECK, SEEN ANY TIME.

"Poor creature," I said. "We'll go around now and buy it." I gave her a look that would curl her. Then I armed her with three crisp pound notes and sent her out to buy a medical book so we'd get all the dope. (I'm beginning to talk like my mother.) Anyhow, she came back hours later with a big dictionary that cost five pounds—she had to expend two of her own—and it has to be seen to be believed, this dictionary. It said things like: "Catarrh, disease of the nostrils."

"Get the preg data," I said, because she's brighter than me in edu-cational matters. She began to read about Fallopian tubes and raised her head from the printed page to tell me she knew a woman who had

two and having two meant you could have two children by two different men at the same time. I was enjoying this, I really was. I took the
book out of her hand and looked up under A for Abortion. They didn't
even consider that word.

"We'll have to get a doctor," she said. "Some nice understanding
doctor."

I couldn't go to the shark down the road that I usually went to,
because he's our family doctor and a Catholic. We got the telephone
book and rang specialists. I'd have paid seventy-five quid, for God's
sake. Well, they had it all so fixed that you had to have appointments
made before you were pregnant—like booking for that Eton lark when
the babies are conceived, before they know whether they'll be cretins
or not—and you had to have a letter from your family doctor. We
thought of friends. She knew someone who knew someone that had a
friend who was a gynecologist. About ten phone calls ensued and the
final one was me talking to this hag who was a lady gynecologist in
the Knightsbridge region. She had one of those voices you hear in
second-class hotels where people are pretending they don't know it's a
second-class hotel.

"Fur example," she said, "aur you bleeding alort?"

"I wish I was," I said. She got very dodgy then and found that her
appointment book was full for an indeterminate time.

"I hope your vowels move tomorrow," I said, and rang off.

"What now?" said Kate, fatalistic. If I hadn't been in such a mess I'd
have said she was sick and ought to be in bed.

"You ought to know someone," I said, "with all your connections";
with her Madame Bovary slop, I thought she'd be adequate to it. "Or
even a crook who'd do a job on a kitchen table in Bayswater," I said.
She gave off a big spiff. How these crooks live a lurid life and make a
fortune by telling about it in the Sunday papers. She said they had little
typists living in terror.

"They can go to hell, they won't get my money," I said in a fit of
sympathy for those goddamn typists, whoever they are.

We went back to the dictionary.

"There's people all over London, happy at this moment, and people
getting on buses, and doing normal things," she said.

"I'll swap them this house and all this gear for it," I said. We were
really low. She had a gray coat on that you could sieve vegetables
through, and her skin was dry like an old cooked potato. Her eyes,
which used to be her good point, were gone back in her head from
crying.

"I'll buy you a coat," I said.

"Did you marry him for money?" she said. I said I didn't know.

"Do you hate him?" she said. I didn't know that, either.

"I don't hate him, I don't love him, I put up with him and he puts up with me," and then I thought of this new disaster and how it would kill his pride, and I got frantic again.

"Baba," she said, "once you have the child, it will be all right. You'll both find it is the most important thing in the world to you. A woman needs children. I'd have more myself."

"Right," said I, "we'll go on a world cruise for our nerves and come back and say 'tis yours."

Boy, did she change her tune. She wasn't ready for children, she said. Who is?

I knew then that it was up to me and I'd better do something, so I told her about the bath and castor-oil plot and asked would she stay, in case I got drowned or had a heart attack. I know she'd really like to have run, but she stayed. I'll say that for her. Not that she was much use. She nearly fainted three times, what with the steam, and the greasy look of the castor oil in the cup, and me sweating and moaning and retching. I had her play "Careless Love" on the record player. She had to go out and put the needle back on that part of the record each time it changed to another song. I thought it was kind of apt.

Suddenly I turned around in my sweating condition and she's kneeling down with her hands joined.

"Get up," I said. "Get up, you lunatic."

"I'm praying," she said. She hadn't said a prayer for years, and even I thought it a bit steep that she should be asking help of someone she'd ignored for so long.

"Nothing short of sacrilege," said I, knowing that would put the wind up her. She was on her feet like lightning, and off to change the needle and put more coal in the boiler. I could hear that boiler roaring up the chimney and I prayed it wouldn't burst or anything until this ordeal was over. He'd kill us. I had cramps and pains, and I began to shake all over. The whole place looked weird. The mirror was all fogged up, and steam all over the place, so that I couldn't see my own makeup and stuff on the various glass racks. I'd look at the hot tap running, then all around, then directly down at the water, hoping to see its color change, then back to the tap again and all around, and I don't know how long I did that.

"Kate, Kate," I said, holding on to the bath as if I was sinking.

"Kate, Kate," I yelled and roared, and she came and said I'd better get out.

"Are you out of your mind?" I said. Imagine going through all the pain and sweat and sickness that I'd gone through and then give up in the middle. I was shaking like a leaf and she held me.

"Good old Florence Nightingale, little old lady with the castor oil," I kept saying, so that she wouldn't think I'd gone too far and call a doctor or do something criminal.

"Jesus," I said suddenly, because it was as if I was stabbed in the butt of my back. I began to howl.

"I'll get brandy," she said.

"Don't leave me, don't leave me," I said. I was dead certain that if she left me I'd fade out. Anyhow, she let go of my arms and I just lolled there, and next thing I know she's giving me brandy from a spoon and saying, "I'm going to phone Frank."

Frank! That revived me. I came to for long enough to say, "If you phone Frank, I'll take twenty-four sleeping pills rights now." She gave me more brandy and turned off the hot tap. I knew as she was turning it off that my chances were over, but I hadn't the energy to resist. The steam, the heat, the castor oil, and then the drink had made me feel like straw. She swears that when I passed out a few seconds later I was a hefty weight to haul out of the bath.

I came to in my own bed with two dressing gowns on me. The first thing I did was to see if anything had resulted, because I'd had a feverish dream that I was in a train and it came, and I couldn't get off the seat, and porters were standing over me yelling at me to get up. Only in the dream had it come.

"Hullo, little old lady with the castor oil," I said to her, sitting there. "T.D.L.," I said, because I was damned if I was going to get all morbid again. No man was worth it.

"Total dead loss," she repeated after me. She was more grave than me.

"We'll get our minks on and hitchhike to the Olympic Games," I said. "I'll enter for the egg-and-spoon race."

She didn't laugh. It was about four o'clock on a lousy afternoon in March, but at least the house was warm because of the way we got the boiler whizzing.

"The gardener came," she said. I could hear him shoveling the snow away. All he could do that winter was shovel snow away so that we could get our Jags in and out, and get up the front steps, drunk, without falling. Not that I'd have minded a fall at that time. It was gray and awful-looking, and I got her to put on the light and draw our sun-drenched blinds.

"Well, it's now for some crook," I said, and pitied those typists again. I was sorry for everyone and no one, the way you are when you're in a mess.

"You can't," she said.

"I go to crooks to have my hair washed," I said. "Where's the difference?"

"The difference is that one is just frivolous, and the other is violence."

Well, Christ, I roared out laughing. I mean, think of being in the state I was, and someone going on like that. Then she launched into a sermon. A whole lot of high-falutin' speech about how I was trying to destroy myself, murder part of myself. A parable, just the way it was in the Gospels. They'd all eat fish and then sit around and hear a story.

Hers was about some woman who was having a baby by a man who loved her, and she didn't want the baby. So she got rid of it. The man stopped loving her, and she fell madly in love with him and went around with a terrible loss in her, because she'd killed two good things.

"But it's not Frank's," I said. As if she didn't know.

"But the point is," she said, "that you don't know beforehand what damage you do to yourself by your actions. You only know afterward."

Well, I couldn't dispute that. I proved it every ten minutes of every day.

"You know her, too," she said.

"What is she like?" said I. There was something about that story that gripped me. I knew I'd be looking out for that woman at the hairdressers.

"We're going to tell Frank," she said, "when he comes in this evening."

"No." I didn't want to tell her the bit about him getting berserk when he got angry. If we told him, there wouldn't be a stick of stuff left in the house, and nothing of me, only bones.

"He'll wreck the joint," I said.

"We'll go to his office," she said. "He can't wreck anything there."

"No," I said.

"Look," she said. She was off again. Another sermon.

The upshot is, I'm dressing myself. She's telling me to put on white makeup and no lipstick and to look wretched. It is not difficult. She'd got me into such a state of righteousness that I was ready to be a suffragette for ten minutes. She said we wouldn't take a car, no, we'd go in all humbleness by bus or Tube. It was miles away in North London. I can tell you, I was pretty wobbly from what was behind me, and from what lay ahead. We damped the boiler, put on our coats, and set out.

Down in the Underground there was a gas advertisement. It said DO NOTHING UNTIL YOU'VE READ VOGUE. Well, in our plight, and with people starving, and having pyorrhea and all sorts of things, I thought it was very vital advice.

"We must come down in the Tube oftener," I said.

"I come every day," she said, making me feel like a rat.

Then a great big enormous pregnant woman appeared from some archway, and that was enough to make me run for the exit stairs.

"Come back, come back," Kate said, catching me by the belt of my camel coat. That minute a Tube tore into the station and she linked me into a No Smoking compartment. We changed into the next compartment at the next station and had a fag each.

"We'll have a few gins along the way," I said. Even she was beginning to lose her fervor.

We got there around four. That was the first time I'd ever been near any of the building sites. They were putting up new blocks of offices on a bomb site, and the ground was snow and yellowish muck. There was an arrow underneath a home-done sign that said INQUIRIES AT OFFICE, and we went in that direction; men booed and whistled at us. Such commotion, such noise hammers clattering and hammering, a great bloody bulldozer churning up more yellow earth, a drill whining and men on the scaffolds yelling in Cockney at Irishmen underneath who couldn't understand a word they were saying. A din. I prayed that the brother wouldn't be with Frank.

"Don't apologize," said Kate, knowing that it was her own worst trait.

"I might funk it in the very middle," I said.

We found him alone in a small, fuggy, little corrugated-iron office with plans and papers laid out all over the table in front of him. He was on the phone.

"Christ," he said when we came in without knocking.

"No, no, Lady Constantine," he said into the phone, "it's just that somebody's capsized a bottle of ink over my notes . . ."

It was about a cesspool that he was going to install in her country cottage. We got bits of the conversation. While she was talking he put his hand over the mouthpiece and said like a savage to Kate, "I hope we haven't to get you out of another mess."

I was kind of glad that I was going to shatter him.

"Yes, it has its own waste-disposal system," he was telling Lady Con, and I knew it was about this cedar-shingled place he'd put up for her in the country. She started on about the roof then. The slates must have been cracking and spalling all over the place. He got red in the face and raised his voice.

"The roof!" he said. "That roof was perfect."

Next thing he was apologizing for his language and saying, "I'll come down there myself."

God help the roof, I thought. He could do a good thousand pounds' worth of damage in five minutes.

"At no cost to you," he said. Then he told her not to worry, and that his bark was worse than his bite. Finally, and after a typical jarvey-driver's farewell, he put the telephone down. Kate stood on my toe just to give me a bit of courage. He didn't look at us for a minute; he wrote some big important nothing into his desk diary and sat there frowning at what he'd written. I could not believe that he was my husband and that I sometimes slept near him and had seen him sick and drunk and in all sorts of conditions. He was another man in that outfit.

"We haven't come about me," said Kate, quite indignant. "We've come to tell you something."

"You'd better make it snappy," he said, "the men knock off at five and we have our conference." He called the men together every evening, and the big, brutal foreman of a brother told who was slacking during the day. Just like the countries we read about where it's supposed to be coercive.

"You tell him." Kate turned to me.

"You begin it," I said.

"It's yours, Baba," she said, very stern. In the end I had to.

"I'm going to have a baby," I said. He grinned, a terrible pathetic grin. It was like telling someone his mother was dead, and you beginning the sentence and he getting it all wrong and thinking his mother had won money. For a minute he thought it was his and that he'd proved himself. He stood up to kiss me, but I put my hand out straightaway. He went like a block of wood; he stayed quite motionless in that position, which is halfway between sitting and standing, and he didn't utter a word. The telephone rang.

"Will I answer it?" I said. He picked it up and threw it, and I ducked, knowing the throwing craze was on. He got more fluent than he'd ever been in his whole life.

"You cow," he said. "There's a way to deal with you and whores like you. I'll kick the arse off you when I get you home."

"I'll take a boat for somewhere," I said.

"You'll do no such thing. You'll bloody well stay where you are and do what you're told."

"Did you think I was going to live frustrated?" I said, just the posh way Kate would say it. I could see he didn't understand that word. There's lots of words like "frustrate" and "masturbate" that he doesn't understand.

"It's not very much for a woman living the way we live," I said. "All that huntin' and shootin' and fishin' lark is all very well in company," I said. He began to close his fist and turn his bottom lip outward, the way he does when he's furious. All this thing about women and new freedom. There isn't a man alive wouldn't kill any woman the minute she draws attention to his defects.

"Watch your language," he said. Boy, it was hot in that room with a double-bar electric heater going full blast!

"I can leave you," I said. "I don't care about a scandal."

He knew of course that it would cause a setback between him and the bishops, and be bad for his work, too, because a lot of the big contracts he got were from Catholic firms.

"I'll tell you what to do," he said.

I could hear heavy footsteps outside crushing their way along the cinder path and I knew that help was arriving. It was the brother to say the meeting was due in a couple of minutes.

"Tell your brother," I said. "He's a great one in a crisis."

The brother killed someone in Ireland once and drove on but was found. They would have jailed him except that he bought his way out.

"Get out," he said, knowing damn well what I meant.

"When I get home there won't be much of you left," he said.

"I won't be there," I said, and wrote the telephone number of Kate's dump on a piece of paper, so that he could ring me if he wanted to.

"What's up?" the brother asked. He has a murderously red face and curly hair.

"The stork," I said as brazen as hell. My knees may have been wobbling under me, but I kept a good front up.

We muddled our way through the muck and got onto the road.

"The eyes of workmen are permanently screwed up; they have to keep them like that in case mortar flies into them," she said. I thought it a boring piece of data, but it got us out of there to the dark street, to bus queues of people.

"Oh no," she said, suddenly defeated. Lucky I had money and could get a taxi to her dump.

"I'll be shacking up with you," I said. "You needn't be lonely anymore."

She looked worried. She's all unnatural about babies and birth.

He rang me about ten. He'd cooled off considerably. He said, "I've decided to let you stay on as my wife—in theory only, of course." Nothing new about that.

"That's great," I said. I suppose he expected a great slob scene from me about how generous and charitable he was. Not me. I know the minute you apologize to people they kill you. Then he wanted to know whose it was so that he could go around and kill him.

"He's a Greek," said I, "and he's gone home."

It was the only thing I could think of. Kate had her head out the bedroom door. She was as inquisitive as hell.

"Will it be white?" said he. The eejit doesn't know Greeks from blacks.

"It might," said I, "if we're lucky." He said he wanted no more cheek from now on and I had to do what I was told and nobody was ever to know the truth.

"Does Brady know?" he said.

"Of course," I said.

"Keep her away from the house. Pay her to keep her bloody mouth shut," he said. He hated her then.

"And go to confession," he said. He then told me he was having a much-deserved holiday to get over the shock, and if anything urgent in the business line arose I was to telephone the secretary.

"Have a nice time," I said, and dashed in to Brady to tell her she could live in elegance with me for a week until he got back.

"It's an ill wind," I said, and she finished the sentence, "that doesn't blow good for someone."

We laughed. A thing we hadn't done for ages.

GLADYS HINDMARCH

from: *A Birth Account* _____

A red heart made of a breadloaf tie sits on my typewriter. It encloses the letters GH. My initials. Cliff. Tied. Thin hairs reach out, he kissed my legs and cunt and bum so gently last night, firm, there, light, his beard stubbles are gruff but his lips are not. My hairs mix with his, reach, stand, wave like cilli, what's the word? those long speary bendy things in the tubes which bring the ovum down, down into the womb.

When he kissed my belly I felt he was kissing both me and you, little one, inside, his love to you direct. That instant I thought you moved to him and I felt you there for the first time, he more with you than I am, how can that be, now I feel you are here, there, I was more afraid of love than he. All three of us are tied in this heart, this belly.

*

Starlings land on the snow-covered compost heap. Through the slit between two apartments, through the thick brown branches of a snow edged tree near the water, a green barge moves. You kick within: light thumps move out slightly in tiny waves. Where you knock doesn't hurt, is slightly like a blood spurt in one spot of a large vein. I smile. Feel soft. The barge moves slowly through the upper-half of the tree. A chunk of snow falls off a telephone wire. I listen to the noonhorns and a dog and a typewriter. And maybe, just maybe, in Herstein's office this afternoon, I'll hear your heart.

*

In a few minutes I'll be swimming in Crystal Pool. Breast stroke is my favorite: arms out, back to the side, together like a heart: breathe, pull, kick, glide. You weigh almost nothing, salt water holds you up, two salt-waters, the one you're in, and the one I'm in. When we're at the pool-ends, I turn slowly, if I don't, you slam my side. Wednesday, 100 turns, 50 lengths in one hour.

*

After fucking last night (which is weird, I get excited but it's not sustained, one second I'm all clitoris, no sensation elsewhere at all, and it's so contained, then we are jumping and bumping around with you between, and I forget, and then I'm a big funny belly with muscles at my back which Cliff bounces on and about), I felt a thin band cross my middle about an inch under surface. It's like a thin chain which jumped lower, shot across and pulled down again. Perhaps this is our first contraction.

*

Driving hurts when I park and unpark. You dont move, but my torso must. Cooking is slower: not at the start but near the finish of each item. Yesterday after I swam, I made potato salad and the last three strokes were so heavy I could hardly get through. Doing anything is longer, elongated, that's a good word: getting up, rinsing a bra, walking to Paul's Meat Market (just half a block along York and a half more down Yew), taking bottles down to the basement, even wiping an ashtray with a serviette is extended: not slower in a clock sense but my rhythms are different, elongated.

ALICE NOTLEY

from: *Songs for the Unborn Second Baby* _____

"Happiness, rage, grief, delight . . . being moved by these passions each
in due degree
        constitutes harmony"
                houses at daybreak, lenses in
oriface, condensed
        watery body a swan—it can only
swim with
        sincerity, warm wine to the heart, effectively
                  archaic
surface of ground trees stones
           light temptation, small light vessels
for rapid moth
        to other planet or bright star
                But we stay
      with our striped petals, raked

      "The second time you get over
              the first"

It was one month behind this one in schedule process that is
As I was five months pregnant that April so am I six
Months pregnant this April and this pregnancy seasonally
Almost imitates the last, except where I was serene thoughtless
In the sweet
      Interruption
         You just
Called me up and I became myself! how mysterious! for I was
Depressed again not my real self you see watch TV
With read endless books beside we make each other, no isolate
Lunacy pools, except sometimes but where was I

Where I was serene thoughtless on the sweet way
In and now I'm hopefully on the way out, from thought
Which is hell, seemed the center of things? of things
Is serenity. Giving birth is cleanly painful what truly
Hurts is learning to live with what you give birth to

BERNADETTE MAYER

from: *The Desires of Mothers to Please Others in Letters*

It finally gets around to the fact there isn't any special breathing you do in labor like duck a l'orange or something, it's labor and you generally pant the midwife said, she said a woman who'd been to some fancy classes wound up saying "out" for fourteen hours, the mantra out. There was a fight at the midwife's between two couples, two fathers were fighting, one was a follower of the guru maharaji and the other was a Biblical Christian, probably born again. The midwife had incidentally said to the wife of the guru that the fetus in the womb goes through all the stages of evolution, now the Biblical man didn't like that and began to excoriate the theory loudly saying that humans were unique and weren't evolved from any kind of other thing and you could prove that by ... and then the guru defensively said he did his Bible-reading too and the midwife said she didn't care, she was a pagan. All this while the midwife was examining the red-haired wife of the guru who seemed to be newly pregnant, then the Biblical couple went in and it seems they were having their fourth child, the woman was enormous and weighed 192 pounds, her baby, due at the same time as mine, a month from now, was also enormous and in her past pregnancies she had had all kinds of problems. Now the Biblical man started being overbearing again and saying why did the problems happen and what could be done to avoid them and the wife was silent, she said her diet was much better than it had been, for some reason the Biblical man was awfully skinny and of course I found myself imagining their fucking, or rather his frenetic fucking with the enormous Biblical woman whom Carol, that's the midwife, was trying to discourage from having her baby at home because of previous complications and the man was saying well this will be her last time so we thought it would be nice to be at home, this man doesn't sound so bad on paper as he was, so anyway there must be an end to his inseminations from the way he had been talking I thought for a while he might have a Biblical stake in endless reproduction, the poor woman. He said he was trying to help with the children, or someone was, because everyone thought the reason for all the woman's problems was having two or three other babies to take care of while she was pregnant and it's true the midwife said you must've had an exhausted uterus which doesn't contract and so she would hemorrhage but then the woman said she hadn't nursed the baby right away and maybe that was the problem, they said they'd been reading up on it. The Biblical man and woman spoke with bad grammar, they were pale and they had pretty children with wide pale faces.

oo oo oo

ANNE WALDMAN

Enceinte _____

Mossy rock, tree limb, foot of a rabbit, large edible root, serpent lashing from side to side, a cushion, veiled lamp, some-kind-of moveable-parts-doll-deity, sponge, rising loaf, butterfly, trapped bird, wax, mold, flame, a small man writing, small woman eating & lifting elbow, a bat, succulent plant, something in the oven, a potato doll, a doll of seashells, sandbag, large fish swimming in circles, a clock, something silent, a silent toy car, a memory, coiled & striking, fish hidden behind rock, every color & no color, a telephone receiver, submarine, rubber expanding, held together with rubber bands, labial, fingers playing an instrument, inflatable doll, a school of dolphins, tidal wave, unease, planet with circling rings, not made in a lab, a thunder storm, lashing out, a chest of toys, sedentary monkey, jack-in-a-box, icebox, lamps going on, a solar system, a tiny city ruled by a cobra, a city of clam inhabitants, an excursion, a place with hats on, an owl, a bear in a cave, drifting raft, boat on the waves, electricity, dancing flame's shadow on your face, bulging package, a rushed person gesturing excitedly as in hailing a speeding taxi cab, quicksilver.

WANDA COLEMAN

Giving Birth _____

against bone. rubbing. pressure against bladder
i pee and pee and pee
and drink water and more water. never enough water
it twists in my womb
my belly a big brown bowl of jello quakes
twenty pounds and climbing
eat eat eat. milk. got to have ice cold milk
vitamins and iron three times daily
cocoa butter and hormone cream
infanstethoscope
sex sex sex. can't get enough of that funky stuff
bras getting too small. is that me in the mirror?
it bucks/brings belches
smooth skin. glossy hair. strong nails
i'm 99% body. my brain has dissolved into
headaches tears confusion
my navel sticks out/eye of cyclops
my life for an apple fritter
snipping the elastic in panties, another pair ruined
nausea. vomit. muscle strain
"they" tell you to eat fresh fruit and lots of
vegetables. eating fresh fruit and lots of vegetables
afraid of what it will/won't be
anxious. it's got to look like him
it's got to look like me. be healthy. be live. be all right
why doesn't it hurry up and come
read books. more books. know the tv program by heart
fantasies about returning to slim
the ass sleeps. tingles when wakened
walking is hard. sitting is hard. sex, an effort
he stands in lines for me
thirty pounds and climbing
people smile, are sympathetic
will it be capricorn or aquarius?
can't drive. too big to get behind the steering wheel
ice cream cone jones
(out of three hundred deliveries this year, ours
is his third legitimate, says doc, "it's what

they are doing to the black community")
daily reports to the grandmothers
is that me in the mirror?
he worries. i worry. we worry together
more hugs and affection
i can't reach my feet
more calcium and iron
wow. my gums are bleeding. scurvy?
it rubs. twists. kicks. moves
sex? it takes too much out of me
the flu. food poisoning. cold
too tight pants bite me
preparation: pelvic spread. vaginal walls widen
forty pounds and climbing
showers. no more long hot luxury baths
muumuus and mules. naked = relief
his ear to my stomach to hear the heart beat
emergency cookies
it presses against my diaphragm. it's hard to
breathe. can't sleep good. dreams
more dreams. it's a boy. it's a girl
backaches. swollen feet
refrigerator lover, clandestine rendezvous at 2 AM
advice from the experienced, questions from the barren
the planets are lining up in scorpio
suitcase packed and ready
names for him. names for her
(everybody-else-we-know-who's-pregnant-is-having
a-perfect-baby pressure)
sex? oh yeah. used to be fun
it turns. kicks. twists
that's me in the mirror, definitely
why doesn't it hurry up and come
crying jags. throb of false labor
will he be there
when it's time?

oo oo oo

BARBARA ROSENTHAL

Baby Moves Inside _____

The baby moves inside my body and Bill reaches for me with his palm open. I think the baby is a boy—two males inside and outside pushing their bodies into mine, moving around me inside and out.

The baby is a girl and Bill reaches for us both, fucks us, loves us both. He kisses my sex, laps at the lips of my vulva where the baby will squeeze through soon, head first, lips first.

Bill waits at my door for his son/daughter, watches, spreads the soft door open trying to catch a glimpse, visiting through the door, reaching in with his cock, knocking at my baby's house. "Are you in there? Who are you? What kind of a person are you?" And the baby responds, knocking back with its tiny feet. "A dancer, an athlete, a person who plants seeds in the ground with my toes."

Does it dream yet? What could it dream about? The days it was a blastocyst? The days I drank a lot of coffee or a little too much wine? (I hope it doesn't remember all those chemical days in the darkroom before I knew it existed—I worry so much ...) Bill pets my curley brown welcome mat, pats my fat tight belly with protruding belly button. "Go back to sleep now," he tells me gently. "We'll make love again in the morning."

ERICA JONG

The Birth of the Water Baby ───────────

Little egg,
little nub,
full complement of
fingers, toes,
little rose blooming
in a red universe,
which once wanted you less
than emptiness,
but now holds you
fast,
containing your rapid heart
beat under its
slower one
as the earth
contains the sea ...

Oh avocado pit
almost ready to sprout,
tiny fruit tree
within sight
of the sea,
little swimming fish,
little land lover,
hold on!
hold on!

Here, under my heart
you'll keep
till it's time
for us to meet,
& we come apart
that we may come
together,
& you are born
remembering
the wavesound
of my blood,

the thunder of my heart,
& like your mother
always dreaming
of the sea.

ON BEING BORN

oo oo oo

LAURA CHESTER

Song of Being Born _____

It was the deepest sleep
It was sleeping in the low note of a big bell
that held and held
I was wrapped in slow motion
wrapped in the fluid gel body a berry sunk down
I opened my eyes it was blurry warm
The feather fern swayed
I'd turn to the steady two-beat pounding
to the rhythm of the blood gong deep distance
Couldn't even feel my skin it was that perfect
in my bag on my back with my hands tossed
over my head that's how I liked it
feet touching soles that how I felt open
Then I'd grip
my cord it throbbed in and out of me
a good thing
to hold it made me connected
and I swung it around my neck as I turned like a scarf
The bowl the bell sleeping sac made me a ball
curled over my shoulders
and settled down
Toes tickled a moss pad my fingers found
lips the little handles on my head but
my head is the bell now
ringing
I feel a pound shift
beginning and it's
different my fluid robe's
torn off
pulled past me sucked into a vacuum I'm
bare in here muscled
The strong stroke is pressing me after
My head stops a cool breeze on the top part plugged
Then rammed
when I was just drifting back to
Rammed against the
this doesn't feel good
My head hurts in circles get heavier

squeezed through a tightness
Can't look now
I've lost it
Just cold and noise and light down the suck hole
Won't give either way
crammed inside
outside it's confusing
Something gripped over my ears hurts metal sounds silver
Like a screech my blood begs
A suction snarl pulling my head off it's
no here come my shoulders
dragged into harshlight
I'm loose I'm so loose they're unwinding my coil scarf
Try to catch it in my hand but
it's cut off a nub I'm cut off
whizzed into space with only small touch points
So bright it hurts so hard I'm going to
fall into the light I'm
feeling for something is surely near
me my mouth says so my lips find fingers want
suck hold *that's it*
I have to suck the light blare
into me
I have to suck the wide space
into me
make me full of warm wash all floating but here's
something wrapped all around with a white tuck
swinging over a milky
place my nose digs for
nuzzles in on what fits it's coming
a lemony sweet warm
shoot on my tongue unfurls
Glom stomp I've found it
where I belong I suck to attach myself a lichen
It's soft too and round too and part of it juts
parts of me and my lips fit
and my body says
alright alright
now suck down
and swallow and go back
to sleep though
never again

that best sleep
that very far back
smooth
sung one

oo oo oo

MARGARET ATWOOD

Giving Birth _____

But who gives it? And to whom is it given? Certainly it doesn't feel like giving, which implies a flow, a gentle handing over, no coercion. But there is scant gentleness here, it's too strenuous, the belly like a knotted fist, squeezing, the heavy trudge of the heart, every muscle in the body tight and moving, as in a slow-motion shot of a high-jump, the faceless body sailing up, turning, hanging for a moment in the air, and then—back to real time again—the plunge, the rush down, the result. Maybe the phrase was made by someone viewing the result only: in this case, the rows of babies to whom birth has occurred, lying like neat packages in their expertly wrapped blankets, pink or blue, with their labels Scotch Taped to their clear plastic cots, behind the plate-glass window.

No one ever says *giving death*, although they are in some ways the same, events, not things. And *delivering*, that act the doctor is generally believed to perform: who delivers what? Is it the mother who is delivered, like a prisoner being released? Surely not; nor is the child delivered to the mother like a letter through a slot. How can you be both the sender and the receiver at once? Was someone in bondage, is someone made free? Thus language, muttering in its archaic tongues of something, yet one more thing, that needs to be re-named.

It won't be by me, though. These are the only words I have, I'm stuck with them, stuck in them. (That image of the tar sands, old tableau in the Royal Ontario Museum, second floor north, how persistent it is. Will I break free, or will I be sucked down, fossilized, a sabre-toothed tiger or lumbering brontosaurus who ventured out too far? Words ripple at my feet, black, sluggish, lethal. Let me try once more, before the sun gets me, before I starve or drown, while I can. It's only a tableau after all, it's only a metaphor. See, I can speak, I am not trapped, and you on your part can understand. So we will go ahead as if there were no problem about language.)

This story about giving birth is not about me. In order to convince you of that I should tell you what I did this morning, before I sat down at this desk—a door on top of two filing cabinets, radio to the left, calendar to the right, these devices by which I place myself in time. I got up at twenty-to-seven, and, halfway down the stairs, met my daughter, who was ascending, autonomously she thought, actually in the arms of her father. We greeted each other with hugs and smiles; we then played with the alarm clock and the hot water bottle, a ritual we go through only on the days her father has to leave the house early to drive into the city. This ritual exists to give me the illusion that I am sleeping in. When she finally decided it was time for me to get up, she began pulling my hair. I got dressed while she explored the bathroom scales and the mysterious white altar of the toilet. I took her downstairs and we had the usual struggle over her clothes. Already she is wearing miniature jeans, miniature T-shirts. After this she fed herself: orange, banana, muffin, porridge.

We then went out to the sun porch, where we recognized anew, and by their names, the dog, the cats and the birds, blue jays and goldfinches at this time of year, which is winter. She puts her fingers on my lips as I pronounce these words; she hasn't yet learned the secret of making them. I am waiting for her first word: surely it will be miraculous, something that has never yet been said. But if so, perhaps she's already said it and I, in my entrapment, my addiction to the usual, have not heard it.

In her playpen I discovered the first alarming thing of the day. It was a small naked woman, made of that soft plastic from which jiggly spiders and lizards and the other things people hang in their car windows are also made. She was given to my daughter by a friend, a woman who does props for movies, she was supposed to have been a prop but she wasn't used. The baby loved her and would crawl around the floor holding her in her mouth like a dog carrying a bone, with the head sticking out one side and the feet out the other. She seemed chewy and harmless, but the other day I noticed that the baby had managed to make a tear in the body with her new teeth. I put the woman into the cardboard box I use for toy storage.

But this morning she was back in the playpen and the feet were gone. The baby must have eaten them, and I worried about whether or not the plastic would dissolve in her stomach, whether it was toxic. Sooner or later, in the contents of her diaper, which I examine with the usual amount of maternal brooding, I knew I would find two small pink plastic feet. I removed the doll and later, while she was still singing to the dog outside the window, dropped it into the garbage. I am not up to finding tiny female arms, breasts, a head, in my daughter's disposable diapers, partially covered by undigested carrots and the husks of raisins, like the relics of some gruesome and demented murder.

Now she's having her nap and I am writing this story. From what I have said, you can see that my life (despite these occasional surprises, reminders of another world) is calm and orderly, suffused with that warm, reddish light, those well-placed blue highlights and reflecting surfaces (mirrors, plates, oblong window-panes) you think of as belonging to Dutch genre paintings; and like them it is realistic in detail and slightly sentimental. Or at least it has an aura of sentiment. (Already I'm having moments of muted grief over those of my daughter's baby clothes which are too small for her to wear any more. I will be a keeper of hair, I will store things in trunks, I will weep over photos.) But above all it's solid, everything here has solidity. No more of those washes of light, those shifts, nebulous effects of cloud, Turner sunsets, vague fears, the impalpables Jeanie used to concern herself with.

I call this woman Jeanie after the song. I can't remember any more of the song, only the title. The point (for in language there are always these "points," these reflections; this is what makes it so rich and sticky, this is why so many have disappeared beneath its dark and shining surface, why you should never try to see your own reflection in it; you will lean over too far, a strand of your hair will fall in and come out gold, and, thinking it is gold all the way down, you yourself will follow, sliding into those outstretched arms, towards the mouth you think is opening to pronounce your name but instead, just before your ears fill with pure sound, will form a word you have never heard before. . . .)

The point, for me, is in the hair. My own hair is not light brown, but Jeanie's was. This is one difference between us. The other point is the dreaming; for Jeanie isn't real in the same way that I am real. But by now, and I mean your time, both of us will have the same degree of reality, we will be equal: wraiths, echoes, reverberations in your own brain. At the moment though Jeanie is to me as I will someday be to you. So she is real enough.

Jeanie is on her way to the hospital, to give birth, to be delivered. She is not quibbling over these terms. She's sitting in the back seat of the car, with her eyes closed and her coat spread over her like a blanket. She is doing her breathing exercises and timing her contractions with a stopwatch. She has been up since two-thirty in the morning, when she took a bath and ate some lime Jell-O, and it's now almost ten. She has learned to count, during the slow breathing, in numbers (from one to ten while breathing in, from ten to one while breathing out) which she can actually see while she is silently pronouncing them. Each number is a different colour and, if she's concentrating very hard, a different typeface. They range from plain roman to ornamented circus numbers, red with gold filigree and dots. This is a refinement not mentioned in any of the numerous books she's read on the subject. Jeanie is a devotee of handbooks. She has at least two shelves of books that cover everything from building kitchen cabinets to auto repairs to smoking your own hams. She doesn't do many of these things, but she does some of them, and in her suitcase, along with a washcloth, a package of lemon Life Savers, a pair of glasses, a hot water bottle, some talcum powder and a paper bag, is the book that suggested she take along all of these things.

(By this time you may be thinking that I've invented Jeanie in order to distance myself from these experiences. Nothing could be further from the truth. I am, in fact, trying to bring myself closer to something that time has already made distant. As for Jeanie, my intention is simple: I am bringing her back to life.)

There are two other people in the car with Jeanie. One is a man, whom I will call A., for convenience. A. is driving. When Jeanie opens her eyes, at the end of every contraction, she can see the back of his slightly balding head and his reassuring shoulders. A. drives well and not too quickly. From time to time he asks her how she is, and she tells him how long the contractions are lasting and how long there is between them. When they stop for gas he buys them each a Styrofoam container of coffee. For months he has helped her with the breathing exercises, pressing on her knee as recommended by the book, and he will be present at the delivery. (Perhaps it's to him that the birth will be given, in the same sense that one gives a performance.) Together they have toured the hospital maternity ward, in company with a small group of other pairs like them: one thin solicitous person, one slow bulbous person. They have been shown the rooms, shared and private, the sitz-baths, the delivery room itself, which gave the impression of being white. The nurse was light-brown, with limber hips and elbows; she laughed a lot as she answered questions.

"First they'll give you an enema. You know what it is? They take a tube of water and put it up your behind. Now, the gentlemen must put on this—and these, over your shoes. And these hats, this one for those with long hair, this for those with short hair."

"What about those with no hair?" says A.

The nurse looks up at his head and laughs. "Oh, you still have some," she says. "If you have a question, do not be afraid to ask."

They have also seen the film made by the hospital, a full-colour film of a woman giving birth to, can it be a baby? "Not all babies will be this large at birth," the Australian nurse who introduces the movie says. Still, the audience, half of which is pregnant, doesn't look very relaxed when the lights go on. ("If you don't like the visuals," a friend of Jeanie's has told her, "you can always close your eyes.") It isn't the blood so much as the brownish-red disinfectant that bothers her. "I've decided to call this whole thing off," she says to A., smiling to show it's a joke. He gives her a hug and says, "Everything's going to be fine."

And she knows it is. Everything will be fine. But there is another woman in the car. She's sitting in the front seat, and she hasn't turned or acknowledged Jeanie in any way. She, like Jeanie, is going to the hospital. She too is pregnant. She is not going to the hospital to give birth, however, because the words, the words, are too alien to her experience, the experience she is about to have, to be used about it at all. She's wearing a cloth coat with checks in maroon and brown, and she has a kerchief tied over her hair. Jeanie has seen her before, but she knows little about her except that she is a woman who did not wish to become pregnant, who did not choose to divide herself like this, who did not choose any of these ordeals, these initiations. It would be no use telling her that everything is going to be fine. The word in English for unwanted intercourse is rape. But there is no word in the language for what is about to happen to this woman.

Jeanie has seen this woman from time to time throughout her pregnancy, always in the same coat, always with the same kerchief. Naturally, being pregnant herself has made her more aware of other pregnant women, and she has watched them, examined them covertly, every time she has seen one. But not every other pregnant woman is this woman. She did not, for instance, attend Jeanie's pre-natal classes at the hospital, where the women were all young, younger than Jeanie.

"How many will be breast-feeding?" asks the Australian nurse with the hefty shoulders.

All hands but one shoot up. A modern group, the new generation, and the one lone bottle-feeder, who might have (who knows?) something wrong with her breasts, is ashamed of herself. The others look politely away from her. What they want most to discuss, it seems, are the differences between one kind of disposable diaper and another. Sometimes they lie on mats and squeeze each other's hands, simulating contractions and counting breaths. It's all very hopeful. The Australian nurse tells them not to get in and out of the bathtub by themselves. At the end of an hour they are each given a glass of apple juice.

There is only one woman in the class who has already given birth. She's there, she says, to make sure they give her a shot this time. They delayed it last time and she went through hell. The others look at her with mild disapproval. *They* are not clamouring for shots, they do not intend to go through hell. Hell comes from the wrong attitude, they feel. The books talk about *discomfort*.

"It's not discomfort, it's pain, baby," the woman says.

The others smile uneasily and the conversation slides back to disposable diapers.

Vitaminized, conscientious, well-read Jeanie, who has managed to avoid morning sickness, varicose veins, stretch marks, toxemia and depression, who has had no aberrations of appetite, no blurrings of vision—why is she followed, then, by this other? At first it was only a glimpse now and then, at the infants' clothing section in Simpson's Basement, in the supermarket lineup, on street corners as she herself slid by in A.'s car: the haggard face, the bloated torso, the kerchief holding back the too-sparse hair. In any case, it was Jeanie who saw her, not the other way around. If she knew she was following Jeanie she gave no sign.

As Jeanie has come closer and closer to this day, the unknown day on which she will give birth, as time has thickened around her so that it has become something she must propel herself through, a kind of slush, wet earth underfoot, she has seen this woman more and more often, though always from a distance. Depending on the light, she has appeared by turns as a young girl of perhaps twenty to an older woman of forty or forty-five, but there was never any doubt in Jeanie's mind that it was the same woman. In fact it did not occur to her that the woman was not real in the usual sense (and perhaps she was, originally, on the first or second sighting, as the voice that causes an echo is real), until A. stopped for a red light during this drive to the hospital and the woman, who had been standing on the corner with a brown paper bag in her arms, simply opened the front door of the car and got in. A. didn't react, and Jeanie knows better than to say anything to him. She is aware that the woman is not really there: Jeanie is not crazy. She could even make the woman disappear by opening her eyes wider, by staring, but it is only the shape that would go away, not the feeling. Jeanie isn't exactly afraid of this woman. She is afraid for her.

When they reach the hospital, the woman gets out of the car and is through the door by the time A. has come around to help Jeanie out of the back seat. In the lobby she is nowhere to be seen. Jeanie goes through Admission in the usual way, unshadowed.

There has been an epidemic of babies during the night and the maternity ward is overcrowded. Jeanie waits for her room behind a dividing screen. Nearby someone is screaming, screaming and mumbling between screams in what sounds like a foreign language. Portuguese, Jeanie thinks. She tells herself that for them it is different, you're supposed to scream, you're regarded as queer if you don't scream, it's a required part of giving birth. Nevertheless she knows that the woman screaming is the other woman and she is screaming from pain. Jeanie listens to the other voice, also a woman's, comforting, reassuring: her mother? A nurse?

A. arrives and they sit uneasily, listening to the screams. Finally Jeanie is sent for and she goes for her prep. Prep school, she thinks. She takes off her clothes—when will she see them again?—and puts on the hospital gown. She is examined, labelled around the wrist and given an enema. She tells the nurse she can't take Demerol because she's allergic to it, and the nurse writes this down. Jeanie doesn't know whether this is true or not but she doesn't want Demerol, she has read the books. She intends to put up a struggle over her pubic hair—surely she will lose her strength if it is all shaved off—but it turns out the nurse doesn't have very strong feelings about it. She is told her contractions are not far enough along to be taken seriously, she can even have lunch. She puts on her dressing gown and rejoins A., in the freshly vacated room, eats some tomato soup and a veal cutlet, and decides to take a nap while A. goes out for supplies.

Jeanie wakes up when A. comes back. He has brought a paper, some detective novels for Jeanie and a bottle of Scotch for himself. A. reads the paper and drinks Scotch, and Jeanie reads *Poirot's Early Cases*. There is no connection between Poirot and her labour, which is now intensifying, unless it is the egg-shape of Poirot's head and the vegetable marrows he is known to cultivate with strands of wet wool (placentae? umbilical cords?). She is glad the stories are short; she is walking around the room now, between contractions. Lunch was definitely a mistake.

"I think I have back labour," she says to A. They get out the handbook and look up the instructions for this. It's useful that everything has a name. Jeanie kneels on the bed and rests her forehead on her arms while A. rubs her back. A. pours himself another Scotch, in the hospital glass. The nurse, in pink, comes, looks, asks about the timing, and goes away again. Jeanie is beginning to sweat. She can only manage half a page or so of Poirot before she has to clamber back up on the bed again and begin breathing and running through the coloured numbers.

When the nurse comes back, she has a wheelchair. It's time to go down to the labour room, she says. Jeanie feels stupid sitting in the wheelchair. She tells herself about peasant women having babies in the fields, Indian women having them on portages with hardly a second thought. She feels effete. But the hospital wants her to ride, and considering the fact that the nurse is tiny, perhaps it's just as well. What if Jeanie were to collapse, after all? After all her courageous talk. An image of the tiny pink nurse, antlike, trundling large Jeanie through the corridors, rolling her along like a heavy beach ball.

As they go by the check-in desk a woman is wheeled past on a table, covered by a sheet. Her eyes are closed and there's a bottle feeding into her arm through a tube. Something is wrong. Jeanie looks back— she thinks it was the other woman—but the sheeted table is hidden now behind the counter.

In the dim labour room Jeanie takes off her dressing gown and is helped up onto the bed by the nurse. A. brings her suitcase, which is not a suitcase actually but a small flight bag, the significance of this has not been lost on Jeanie, and in fact she now has some of the apprehensive feelings she associates with planes, including the fear of a crash. She takes out her Life Savers, her glasses, her washcloth and the other things she thinks she will need. She removes her contact lenses and places them in their case, reminding A. that they must not be lost. Now she is purblind.

There is something else in her bag that she doesn't remove. It's a talisman, given to her several years ago as a souvenir by a travelling friend of hers. It's a rounded oblong of opaque blue glass, with four yellow-and-white eye shapes on it. In Turkey, her friend has told her, they hang them on mules to protect against the Evil Eye. Jeanie knows this talisman probably won't work for her, she is not Turkish and she isn't a mule, but it makes her feel safer to have it in the room with her. She had planned to hold it in her hand during the most difficult part of labour but somehow there is no longer any time for carrying out plans like this.

An old woman, a fat old woman dressed all in green, comes into the room and sits beside Jeanie. She says to A., who is sitting on the other side of Jeanie, "That is a good watch. They don't make watches like that any more." She is referring to his gold pocket watch, one of his few extravagances, which is on the night table. Then she places her hand on Jeanie's belly to feel the contraction. "This is good," she says, her accent is Swedish or German. "This, I call a contraction. Before, it was nothing." Jeanie can no longer remember having seen her before. "Good. Good."

"When will I have it?" Jeanie asks, when she can talk, when she is no longer counting.

The old woman laughs. Surely that laugh, those tribal hands, have presided over a thousand beds, a thousand kitchen tables ... "A long time yet," she says. "Eight, ten hours."

"But I've been *doing* this for twelve hours already," Jeanie says.

"Not hard labour," the woman says. "Not good, like this."

Jeanie settles into herself for the long wait. At the moment she can't remember why she wanted to have a baby in the first place. That decision was made by someone else, whose motives are now unclear. She remembers the way women who had babies used to smile at one another, mysteriously, as if there was something they knew that she didn't, the way they would casually exclude her from their frame of reference. What was the knowledge, the mystery, or was having a baby really no more inexplicable than having a car accident or an orgasm? (But these too were indescribable, events of the body, all of them; why should the mind distress itself trying to find a language for them?) She has sworn she will never do that to any woman without children, engage in those passwords and exclusions. She's old enough, she's been put through enough years of it to find it tiresome and cruel.

But—and this is the part of Jeanie that goes with the talisman hidden in her bag, not with the part that longs to build kitchen cabinets and smoke hams—she is, secretly, hoping for a mystery. Something more than this, something else, a vision. After all she is risking her life, though it's not too likely she will die. Still, some women do. Internal bleeding, shock, heart failure, a mistake on the part of someone, a nurse, a doctor. She deserves a vision, she deserves to be allowed to bring something back with her from this dark place into which she is now rapidly descending.

She thinks momentarily about the other woman. Her motives, too, are unclear. Why doesn't she want to have a baby? Has she been raped, does she have ten other children, is she starving? Why hasn't she had an abortion? Jeanie doesn't know, and in fact it no longer matters why. *Uncross your fingers*, Jeanie thinks to her. Her face, distorted with pain and terror, floats briefly behind Jeanie's eyes before it too drifts away.

Jeanie tries to reach down to the baby, as she has many times before, sending waves of love, colour, music, down through her arteries to it, but she finds she can no longer do this. She can no longer feel the baby as a baby, its arms and legs poking, kicking, turning. It has collected itself together, it's a hard sphere, it does not have time right now to listen to her. She's grateful for this because she isn't sure anyway how good the message would be. She no longer has control of the numbers either, she can no longer see them, although she continues mechanically to count. She realizes she has practised for the wrong thing, A. squeezing her knee was nothing, she should have practised for this, whatever it is.

"Slow down," A. says. She's on her side now, he's holding her hand. "Slow it right down."

"I can't, I can't do it, I can't do this."

"Yes, you can."

"Will I sound like that?"

"Like what?" A. says. Perhaps he can't hear it: it's the other woman, in the room next door or the room next door to that. She's screaming and crying, screaming and crying. While she cries she is saying, over and over, "It hurts. It hurts."

"No, you won't," he says. So there is someone, after all.

A doctor comes in, not her own doctor. They want her to turn over on her back.

"I can't," she says. "I don't like it that way." Sounds have receded, she has trouble hearing them. She turns over and the doctor gropes with her rubber-gloved hand. Something wet and hot flows over her thighs.

"It was just ready to break," the doctor says. "All I had to do was touch it. Four centimetres," she says to A.

"Only *four?*" Jeanie says. She feels cheated; they must be wrong. The doctor says her own doctor will be called in time. Jeanie is outraged at them. They have not understood, but it's too late to say this and she slips back into the dark place, which is not hell, which is more like being inside, trying to get out. *Out*, she says or thinks. Then she is floating, the numbers are gone, if anyone told her to get up, go out of the room, stand on her head, she would do it. From minute to minute she comes up again, grabs for air.

"You're hyperventilating," A. says. "Slow it down." He is rubbing her back now, hard, and she takes his hand and shoves it viciously further down, to the right place, which is not the right place as soon as his hand is there. She remembers a story she read once, about the Nazis tying the legs of Jewish women together during labour. She never really understood before how that could kill you.

A nurse appears with a needle. "I don't want it," Jeanie says.

"Don't be hard on yourself," the nurse says. "You don't have to go through pain like that." What pain? Jeanie thinks. When there is no pain she feels nothing, when there is pain, she feels nothing because there is no *she*. This, finally, is the disappearance of language. *You don't remember afterwards*, she has been told by almost everyone.

Jeanie comes out of a contraction, gropes for control. "Will it hurt the baby?" she says.

"It's a mild analgesic," the doctor says. "We wouldn't allow anything that would hurt the baby." Jeanie doesn't believe this. Nevertheless she is jabbed, and the doctor is right, it is very mild, because it doesn't seem to do a thing for Jeanie, though A. later tells her she has slept briefly between contractions.

Suddenly she sits bolt upright. She is wide awake and lucid. "You have to ring that bell right now," she says. "This baby is being born."

A. clearly doesn't believe her. "I can feel it, I can feel the head," she says. A. pushes the button for the call bell. A nurse appears and checks, and now everything is happening too soon, nobody is ready. They set off down the hall, the nurse wheeling Jeanie feels fine. She watches the corridors, the edges of everything shadowy because she doesn't have her glasses on. She hopes A. will remember to bring them. They pass another doctor.

"Need me?" she asks.

"Oh no," the nurse answers breezily. "Natural childbirth."

Jeanie realizes that this woman must have been the anaesthetist.

"What?" she says, but it's too late now, they are in the room itself, all those glossy surfaces, tubular strange apparatus like a science-fiction movie, and the nurse is telling her to get onto the delivery table. No one else is in the room.

"You must be crazy," Jeanie says.

"Don't push," the nurse says.

"What do you mean?" Jeanie says. This is absurd. Why should she wait, why should the baby wait for them because they're late?

"Breathe through your mouth," the nurse says. "Pant," and Jeanie finally remembers how. When the contraction is over she uses the nurse's arm as a lever and hauls herself across onto the table.

From somewhere her own doctor materializes, in her doctor suit already, looking even more like Mary Poppins than usual, and Jeanie says, "Bet you weren't expecting to see me so soon!" The baby is being born when Jeanie said it would, though just three days ago the doctor said it would be at least another week, and this makes Jeanie feel jubilant and smug. Not that she knew, she'd believed the doctor.

She's being covered with a green tablecloth, they are taking far too long, she feels like pushing the baby out now, before they are ready. A. is there by her head, swathed in robes, hats, masks. He has forgotten her glasses. "Push now," the doctor says. Jeanie grips with her hands, grits her teeth, face, her whole body together, a snarl, a fierce smile, the baby is enormous, a stone, a boulder, her bones unlock, and, once, twice, the third time, she opens like a birdcage turning slowly inside out.

A pause; a wet kitten slithers between her legs. "Why don't you look?" says the doctor, but Jeanie still has her eyes closed. No glasses, she couldn't have seen a thing anyway. "Why don't you look?" the doctor says again.

Jeanie opens her eyes. She can see the baby, who has been wheeled up beside her and is fading already from the alarming birth purple. A good baby, she thinks, meaning it as the old woman did: *a good watch*, well-made, substantial. The baby isn't crying; she squints in the new light. Birth isn't something that has been given to her, nor has she taken it. It was just something that has happened so they could greet each other like this. The nurse is stringing beads for her name. When the baby is bundled and tucked beside Jeanie, she goes to sleep.

As for the vision, there wasn't one. Jeanie is conscious of no special knowledge; already she's forgetting what it was like. She's tired and very cold; she is shaking, and asks for another blanket. A. comes back to the room with her; her clothes are still there. Everything is quiet, the other woman is no longer screaming. Something has happened to her, Jeanie knows. Is she dead? Is the baby dead? Perhaps she is one of those casualties (and how can Jeanie herself be sure, yet, that she will not be among them) who will go into postpartum depression and never come out. "You see, there was nothing to be afraid of," A. says before he leaves, but he was wrong.

The next morning Jeanie wakes up when it's light. She's been warned about getting out of bed the first time without the help of a nurse, but she decides to do it anyway (peasant in the field! Indian on the portage!). She's still running adrenaline, she's also weaker than she thought, but she wants very much to look out the window. She feels she's been inside too long, she wants to see the sun come up. Being awake this early always makes her feel a little unreal, a little insubstantial, as if she's partly transparent, partly dead.

(It was to me, after all, that the birth was given, Jeanie gave it, I am the result. What would she make of me? Would she be pleased?)

The window is two panes with a venetian blind sandwiched between them; it turns by a knob at the side. Jeanie has never seen a window like this before. She closes and opens the blind several times. Then she leaves it open and looks out.

All she can see from the window is a building. It's an old stone building, heavy and Victorian, with a copper roof oxidized to green. It's solid, hard, darkened by soot, dour, leaden. But as she looks at this building, so old and seemingly immutable, she sees that it's made of water. Water, and some tenuous jelly-like substance. Light flows through it from behind (the sun is coming up), the building is so thin, so fragile, that it quivers in the slight dawn wind. Jeanie sees that if the building is this way (a touch could destroy it, a ripple of the earth, why has no one noticed, guarded it against accidents?) then the rest of the world must be like this too, the entire earth, the rocks, people, trees, everything needs to be protected, cared for, tended. The enormity of this task defeats her; she will never be up to it, and what will happen then?

Jeanie hears footsteps in the hall outside her door. She thinks it must be the other woman, in her brown-and-maroon-checked coat, carrying her paper bag, leaving the hospital now that her job is done. She has seen Jeanie safely through, she must go now to hunt through the streets of the city for her next case. But the door opens, it's a nurse, who is just in time to catch Jeanie as she sinks to the floor, holding on to the edge of the air-conditioning unit. The nurse scolds her for getting up too soon.

After that the baby is carried in, solid, substantial, packed together like an apple, Jeanie examines her, she is complete, and in the days that follow Jeanie herself becomes drifted over with new words, her hair slowly darkens, she ceases to be what she was and is replaced, gradually, by someone else.

LYN LIFSHIN

North _____

feels the seal fur
wetting under her the
smell of burning

blood digs into
a bracelet of ivory the
black hair bursts out
from her thighs

trembling nothing
else cuts the blue

stillness the other
women melt snow
the moon touches the
baby's tiny penis

she falls back in a
dream of water
placenta buried in
the earth floor

safe from animals
unbilical cord in a
caribou skull

to bring sun
and joy to
both of them

oo oo oo

MAXINE CHERNOFF

A Birth _____

> *"We must seek bodies for our children."*
> —*Osage Indian chant*

I can't remember the birth. Cold white rooms, cleanliness
the color of nothing. Sometimes a woman dreams that she's
given birth to a litter of piglets attached to her breasts like
pink balloons. When I look in the crib there is no baby;
when I look on the stove there is a pot of soup which was not
there before. Sometimes there is a mix-up at the hospital. A
patient orders French onion soup and receives cream of
shrimp. Sometimes there is a mix-up; a woman receives a
child who grows up hating her. One night at a theatre a
person walks out of the screen and sits down beside her.
That is her child, she knows. "The soup is ready," my
husband repeats. Silently we sit down side by side. Silently
we share one bowl.

DAPHNE MARLATT

Rings, iv. _____

Eyes shut. Relax now, can relax all over, breathe like
asleep, pretend to be sleeping if you can remember how it
feels, whole, your whole body, before it comes again. But
don't think of that now, relax. Al, listen, Al's still reading,

> *'I beg your pardon,' the doctor said. 'I am perhaps*
> *a little jealous since you use your language to communicate*
> *with yourself and not with us ...'*
>   (can't get comfortable,
To relax. Wrong side maybe.)
>   *'I do my art in both languages,'*
> *Deborah said, but she did not miss the threat ...*

                                        (oh there's
the sheet, the, Beginning to tighten now, lie still, Relax
everything but that, now, A breathing, climb, higher, B,
breathe higher, C, it's all turning to, liquid, hot, spasm
(smother), OH, very deep in, all, in it grinding me to liquid
shit again ... shit.

                    Up. Al: again? Can't help it. That damn
enema. And that i ASKED for it, thinking it would rid me of
this feeling, this, terrible urge to go, got to, hurry (totter)
down the hall in this, ridiculous, gown. I feel like a child
half out of clothes, bare back cool. To get there before (ah,
this long corridor almost normal, window, life goes on out
there's a busy day, traffic
                        Here. The door & tiled floor under
my feet, won't turn on the light it's so small & stuffy in here.
Sit, thank god, but now (crack of light under the door) if only
it would all come out. But what if i had the baby in the toilet,
in the dark. If i could just curl up on the floor there's not
even enough room (bet they made it like this on purpose) maybe
it's a natural urge just to curl up in the dark on my own (cats
do it) on my own i could be calm. Here it comes, relax (how
can i relax on the toilet? should be back in bed) why did i
come? You should have known there was nothing more. Stop
thinking of that now, too late, breathe,

It's tighter, breathe higher,
Oh, hands against the walls, hang on, no, let go, go into it,
don't fight it (all doubled up) don't fall into the toilet.
LET GO. Oh, that was bad. Hardly breathed at all. 'Cause you
were scared. Scared of being alone when it happened, when
something happened. After all that about the dark. Better go
back before it comes again.

Down the hall. There he is, the
doctor, such a small man, owl man, & so imperious. But he
does look worried. Where were you? Now don't get up again.
You're not supposed to be wandering around after the waters
break.

Little girl being scolded. But he was actually
concerned. Al in that silly gown ushers me in. They couldn't
believe you'd gone to the bathroom. Nobody told me not to.
I know, but you don't have to go anymore, you can't possibly
HAVE anymore. But it FEELS like it.

Nurse pops in. Do you
want some demerol? The doctor said you could have some. Like
it was a gift.
No.

Up on the bed again (up on the roof, might
as well be.) With a little help (getting weak? feeling
well worked, sweaty). Now, find the right position. Because,
is it? Yes, it's coming again. Relax, breathe. Good, i'll
do it this time, i'll ride over it. Breathe higher. Remember
to relax everything. That leg too. Higher, faster, But it's
bearing down, Harder, not the right position, it's going to,
suck me in, quick, think of what Al's reading.

*By the light of
my fire, Bird-one, Anterrabae said* (breathe) *see how carefully, how carefully* (higher) *they separate you from small
dangers* (pant) : *pins and matches and belts and shoelaces
and dirty looks.* (It's going.) *Will Ellis beat the naked
witness in a locked seclusion room?*
Where is that?
a third of the way through? I can't remember. Wonder how long
it's been. Seems a long time i've been turning, twisting, half

the sheets on the floor. There must be some way, some position.
What did the book say for back labour? Try it on your side,
face Al, the book, the sunny window. sunny. Now relax. It's
not pain, it crushes me, it grinds me into thick, hot, water.
it wears me down fighting it. If i could only, let go.

. . .

I've settled into it. Tired & floaty warm. Except my feet
are cold, Did they say that? your feet will be cold. Al's
socks, & my legs all bristly, i didn't shave. Well it doesn't
matter, i can't get into that. Socks feel good.

Why couldn't i eat the soup? It smelled meaty, nourishing.
Chicken noodle. such work to eat the noodles. even the broth.
But the red jello they brought (& i spilled, sticky against
my leg), so cold & clear, sweet. like sun in Jim's wine glass
that time in nashville when the day stood still, all that
afternoon was dust in everything we ate, luminous, air
thick with it like pollen/honey moved thru, always, never
notice. Coming, & it doesn't matter, i can ride it. be a
cat relaxed & lie so it contracts but doesn't move me,
stays, limbs dissociated while it, breathe higher, grinds
my belly, back, to liquid, panting's a familiar place
at work, it's going, it does work, the breathing does . . .

'*Well, really, every* CASE *like you ought to realize that*
THAT HELL'—*and she began to shake with shudders of high
shrill laughter*—'*can't last any more than you can stand it.
It's like physical pain*—*tee-hee-hee*—*there's just so much
and then, no* MORE.'

            It doesn't matter. He's right, or she is.
But i'm not the same as them, which seems so far away i can't
get into it. He is, though. I've never heard him read aloud
a drama, personalities. strange world. Strange book, but that's
all right, he's reading it to me. What was the book we were
going to? or the song we never did decide. Now it comes,
they said god save the queen if you want, higher now, i never
seem to need it, just climb higher, panting, feel it clench
deep, still the ends of me relax. panic's gone. Why didn't i
take demerol before?
            This could go on all afternoon, Al reading,

my warm sticky bed, sun thru the window, i know it's sunny
out there, afternoon, could go on for hours tho the hours lead
somewhere, lead me, i don't fight to get there. Is he really
into the book? I might tell him, but it doesn't matter,
let his voice move on. I feel warm & tired, catlike. Even
the blood trickling down is comfortable. it's me. it's
happening as if i KNEW how it would be.

Uuungh. Against the wall, push my arm against the wall &
push it thru my arm, that terrible urge to convulse, push,
get it out. No, it's a mistake, you're not ready yet, you
could hurt yourself. Don't push. I WANT TO twist my body
against it. want to constrict. Stay open, open. against
this WRINGING? It comes so fast, i've got to, got to. Don't.
And rigid, all my relaxation gone beyond it, hold the
pelvic floor loose & work it thru your arms,

                                    Uuungh, it's not
pain, it's got to, got to. that FORCE. I want to scream i
give up, twist into one tight fist, clench, & push it,
PUSH it.

       You're doing fine.

                       Ha. Why don't they let me?
You know why. Al, folding my arm & saying one two blow. He's
doing it too fast, but he remembered, he's doing it. Not yet.
Yet, yes, blow, blow. The book said you can't blow & push
at the same time. Blooow. You can. i still did. Don't.
Everything's speeding up. One, two, blowowow.

                             There's only a
little bit left, hang in there.

                As if i can, as if i will it!
They don't know. Can't hang on much longer, going to, the
next one, going to give in. Oh now, blow. Try. You might
hurt his head. Blow. There's the sponge (Al) on my lips.
Can't open my eyes to thank him. Coming again. Ah, ah, can't
stop it, stop writhing around & pushing.

                    That did it,
the nurse said, that was the worst one, the others won't
be so bad.

And they're wheeling me out, it's happening. The open door.

. . .

A lot of people in gowns & they're all talking busy. A lot of white light. A table they slide me onto & there's the doctor, Well, smile. after all this we're ready! & the anaesthetist (? yes) & someone saying, Oh she's fine, she's doing very well. Can't answer. It's coming. Push. Again, push. Was i really pushing? It didn't seem to be pushing from inside.

And there's the mirror where i can see, except he's standing in the way. They've got me all positioned, knees up, feet in stirrups (fear, a bit). Al's at my head. There's so much going on i can't follow. so much talk. It's coming again, now push. Now someone's saying push. hard. that's still not hard enough. Going to have hemorrhoids tomorrow, all that blood rushing into my face.

I look up at Al behind the mask, his eyes look encouraging. Next time i'll be ready for it. & someone's saying, You can really push now, give it all you've got. I'm not doing it right. But it's so hard to tell when it begins & then it's here & i'm left behind, pushing, no. block & push. push. Too late, the tail end.

A shot? No, no, it's just salts. your blood pressure's high. Well at least i'm working, even if it doesn't feel right. But this time, this time i'm ready & remember, it's the blocking, build up pressure &, time it just right to (push), block &

PUSH . . .

Nothing's different. There in the mirror hardly any hole, just a little dark space. Why doesn't it change? How long has she been listening to his heart with the stethoscope? Something's wrong? Again now. Block &, push, PUSH. And the doctor's saying, We're going to use forceps, he's posterior. What's that again? face up? he's supposed to be face down? He's lying relaxing with his hands behind his head, he says. Relaxing?! Little person.

And the anaesthetist is kind in
explaining what the epidural will do, what it will knock out.
The least, i say, i want the least. & the doctor: it's what's
best for the baby, he's getting tired. You don't have to
remind me, i want to say, i want him healthy, whole. of
course it's for him, whatever you say. & to the anaesthetist,
who is young & seems sympathetic, Will i still feel him?
You will feel something but you won't feel as much as you
would ordinarily, & you won't feel the episiotomy. Yes, well
(that's not important). & they give it to me. & now he's
standing with Al drawing diagrams on my pillow of the nerves
which are getting knocked out. I can't feel the contraction,
the nurse has her hand at the top of my belly, she has to
tell me, now PUSH. & i push by sheer will because i can't
feel my muscles pushing down there, but i push. & it's a
good push. Someone said, there's a lock of dark hair. i keep
thinking, dark hair. Has he cut me yet? can i see? Whenever
i open my eyes the room is filled with white bustling,
everyone doing something specific. we're all working together
for him, for this one with his hands behind his head who
doesn't even know. When i look in the mirror it's much wider,
there IS hair. His hair! all matted against my red flesh.
Now lie back. & i feel the forceps go in, barely. There's
the head, they say. Now gently, now hardly push at all.
& i feel something like a loss, like the end of a sigh,
A cry! a squall of absolute protest, pain? He's real. &
i haven't seen him! & someone says a boy (i knew) with
black hair. They lay the cord on my stomach & he's upside
down, streaked with blood, & reddish, his small round buttocks
& head all wet, matted, all that hair. They turn him, such
big balls.
   He's crying. I can't stand it, i want to hold him,
PLEASE. & they lay him snuggled in a blanket on my stomach.
He's perfect, bawling, little blue fists. small & perfectly
HERE. He's here, i say to Al. & he's beautiful. Al's
bending over, a little shy but grinning too. & he is,
& i say to everybody, he's beautiful. Most of all to him,
because he's come thru that ring of flesh, into our light,
he's BORN, tight fisted in my arms, eyes screwed shut,
shutting us out. Yet he can hear & maybe feel someone
cradling him against her, hush. hush. i hold him. it's
all right. you're born.

DEENA METZGER

from: *Skin: Shadows/Silence* _____

And when she was ready to deliver, she let him hold her legs, and he pressed down harshly on her stomach and with a grunt, forced the child squalling between her legs.

And when she was ready to deliver, she spread her legs from one post to another in front of all her friends who had come together not for a birth but for a death; she slit her belly up the middle with a paring knife and pulled out the bloody child.

And when she was ready to deliver, they pulled her into a white room and tied her legs to the table and a man she had never met before thrust his hairy but gloved arm into her vaginal passage and made a fist about the head and pulled out the bloody child.

And when she was ready to deliver, she went to a pool of water by herself and let the waves break upon her with each contraction, so the child was born into the sea and shone with brine.

And when she was ready to deliver, he was torn as to which one to save and he saw the head between her legs in the very spot where he had drunk and his first instinct was to run because he wanted neither of them if he could not have each alone but finally because she was in such pain and he could not bear to see her body heaving in contractions desperate to expel the child which could not break out by itself, he put his hand almost it seemed to him entirely within her womb, and with fear and gentleness urged the child out. He didn't notice how covered he was with her blood when he wrapped the child in his shirt against the cold and then he closed her legs upon the pain.

It is possible, she said, to nurse an infant with one breast and to put the other breast in the father's mouth. And all the dreams shuffle from one mouth to the other. And the milk runs thin as sperm.

And when she was ready to deliver, he confirmed his desire to deliver the child and lay down beside her. During intense moments of pain, he held her hand, rubbed her belly, pushed and groaned with her. The pain invaded his body like an electric current, passing from her to him and when he felt it, he stiffened so as to absorb most of it and hold it without allowing it to pass back into her. She, however, was unwilling to let him bear it all. It was her child and she wanted to feel it born. But it was his child and he also wanted to be rent by it. It was selfishness then that caused them to fight with each other for the birth pains. And the child was born almost without their noticing it. And he had not taken his eyes from his wife's face. The pain brought tears to her eyes. She was pale, exhausted. Her hair was stringy with sweat.

At the last moment he pressed his palms over her entire body in order to imbed the memory of pregnancy in his hands. "We haven't had enough time," he said. And they were both naked. He felt the last contraction on his skin and the child slipped out of both of them.

It cried as soon as it was born and he kissed the baby on the mouth and then kissed her and pushed his tongue into her mouth so they were joined again. And the child cried lustily.

> *If a woman have conceived seed, and born a man child: then she shall be unclean seven days;*
>
> *And she shall then continue in the blood of her purifying three and thirty days; she shall touch no hallowed thing, nor come into the sanctuary, until the days of her purifying be fulfilled.*
>
> *But if she bear a maid child, then she shall be unclean two weeks;*
>
> *And she shall continue in the blood of her purifying three score and six days.*
>
> *And when the days of her purifying are fulfilled, for a son, or for a daughter, she shall bring a lamb of the first year for a burnt offering, and a young pigeon, or a turtledove, for a sin offering, unto the door of the tabernacle of the congregation, unto the priest.*

o o   o o   o o

SHARON DOUBIAGO

from: South America Mi Hija _____

She took my clothes, put me
on that hard board in that tiny green cell,
tied a paper to my neck.
He sat at my feet. Silent. But there.
An occasional grin. The consummate moment
of our teenage marriage.
I had always been told I was beautiful
which made me ugly.
Now I was beautiful.
In the bursting of your coming, muscle, skin, walls,
the smock untied. I leaned back on my hands,
my stretched, engorged breasts exposed, laughed,
entered a strange stream, a sexual
stream, the ecstasy of time and place, a churning
like mountains, like seas at the risen continents.
I could hear time, a machine sound.
I could feel creation, myself in place
for the first time.

SUMMER BRENNER

Whithertofore _____

Annie walked along. Feeling relieved. She had let him
have it. That was good. And she hoped it ruined his afternoon. She
stopped at a stationery store. Picked up a small box of pastels and a
drawing pad and made her way to the bus stop. Most of the small
shops had closed, and the town was quiet with lunch and siesta.

The streets stank with diesel exhaust. Annie found the #19 and got
on. There were just a few people. Late going home for the mid-day
meal. Two large dark women with a child. An old man with eyes full
of God and cataracts. As if a diseased vision brought him closer to the
sight of his soul. And a very young and handsome man. Dark and
round-featured. Looked Indian.

Annie sat a few seats behind him looking directly at the back of his
neck. And his lavender shirt. His neck was large without being dumb.
Husky. Hunky. Stocky. Chunky. He definitely had a mass to him she
liked. He was probably a fisherman.

The bus roared off through the center and on to the outskirts of
town. It cut west and suddenly the bay was straight ahead in full view.
The bus jostled its way past huts and banana trees. The village was
about 12 miles south. Annie looked out the window. The flashing
clotheslines. The curious children. The buzzards clinging to some mo-
torized carcass. Something about this jungle that was so gorgeous. Always half-decayed.

Martin and her mood had passed. She was out now. And it was an
adventure.

The land was a hotline to New Mexico. In exact opposition. The
desert and the jungle. Living between the mesas and the rocks. Among
the muted mercurial browns. It was the perfect complement to the
gaudy vines. Laura way back there on the mountain with her two goats
and new baby. And her here on a rickety bus in a garden of succulents.

Laura's labor time had been average for a first baby. 15 hours. She
had had her boy at home, and Annie had been there. The first few
hours had been hilarious. Laura said if Annie didn't stop making her
laugh, she was never going to have that baby. By 3 a.m. things were a
lot more serious.

Laura had constant pain in her back, and Annie and Alan and the
midwife took turns pressing down on the coccyx to relieve the pressure.
She let the long moans come out from her belly. Thank God they

hadn't been in a hospital. They probably would have insisted on using a needle. One thing the natural childbirth books said was that you had to be cool in a hospital situation. Or at least sound cool. Laura absented herself from her body to get through the pain.

Beliefs about childbirth were really confused. What was that horror story. About a midwife in California who had been arrested by one of her patients. A pregnant undercover cop. At least in New Mexico midwifery was still legal.

Part of it surely was greed. Doctors. They had spent so many years in school learning more about sickness than health. Tom had gone to Harvard, and he said his teachers talked about *the hands*. The laying on of hands. The importance of healing as well as curing. Most schools weren't like that. And neither were doctors.

Annie's own first visit to a gynecologist had been painless and cold. The stirrups. The rubber gloves. The nurse in the room. They said that was to make sure the doctor could never be accused of rape.

Laura let the long sounds come. Contractions every forty seconds. Laura wanting to get out of bed. She stood up and the waters broke. The amniotic sack. A pool of skim milk all over the floor. Then she said she couldn't go on. We were holding her hands. She sank down to the floor. Thirty minutes later William Everett Bumper Jack Tire Truck Prince of the Rodeo Pea Pod was born. Now that was beautiful.

Laura just got up and took a shower. Sat on the bed with Alan and ate chicken and drank champagne.

Being in Mexico made Annie want to fill herself up like a fruit. Until she burst.

The bus had stopped. There it was. The typical. The quaint. The predictable. The picturesque. The beautiful quiet lazy town. San Lucas del Mar.

oo oo oo
NIKKI GIOVANNI

from: Don't Have a Baby till You Read This ____

The nurses all said, "You're fine now, Mother," and I said, "My name is Nikki," and they said, "Yes, Mother." So when Gary came I was interested in how I had done. And she, typical of hospital personnel, said, "You're much better now." So I said, "How was I then?" "A good patient." And I said, "Gary, when I get up I'm gonna kill you if you don't tell me." "Well, you would have come through with flying colors if your heart hadn't stopped. That gave the doctors some concern for a while. Then the baby—he's cute; did you know he was sucking his thumb in the incubator? The smartest little guy back there. Well, he was lying on your bladder and a piece of it came out. But other than that you're fine. Mommy and Gus and Barb and I were with you all the time." And I thought, uh-huh. "And Chris is really glad you had a boy. He said he knew you could do it if you wanted." And I thought, uh-huh.

Then she had to leave the floor because the babies were coming. I pulled my gown straight and worked my way into a sitting position and smiled warmly like mothers are supposed to do. And the girl next to me got her baby. Then all the people on my side. Then all the people on the other side. And I started to cry. The floor nurse said, "What's the matter, Mother?" and I cried, "Something has happened to my baby and nobody will tell me about it." And she said, "No. Nursery didn't know you were well. I'll go get it for you." And I said, "Him. It's a boy." So she brought you to me and Gary was right. Undoubtedly the most beautiful, intelligent, everything baby in the world. You had just finished eating so we sat, you in your bassinet and me in my bed, side by side. Then the nurse said, "Don't you want to hold him?" And I started to say, bitch, holding is to mothers what sucking is to babies what corners are to prostitutes what evasion is to politicians. But I just looked at her and she looked at the lines into and out of me so she put you in the bed, and you were very quiet because you knew I didn't feel too swell and if you did anything I wouldn't be able to help you.

The next morning my doctor came by and said his usual and I said, "I guess so I'm alive," and he said, "If you'll eat I'll take the tube out of your arm." Remembering what hospital food had been like when I'd had my hemorrhoidectomy a couple of years back, I hesitated, but he reminded me that I could feed you so I was suckered. And I was glad because I met the dietician, who was really a wonderful woman. But I made the mistake of saying I liked oatmeal and she made the mistake of giving me a lot and I didn't eat it, and they said, "Mother, if you don't eat we'll have to put the tube back in." So I had to tell her to keep my diet thing together. Institutions make it hard for you to make friends. Then someone asked if I wanted you circumcised and I said yes and they brought you back and you were maaaad. And I loved it because you showed a lot of spirit. And I snuck you under the covers and we went to sleep because we'd both had a long, hard day. They said you wouldn't let the nurse in white touch you for a good long time after that, which is what I dig about you—you carry grudges. And that was a turning point. I decided to get you out of there before they got your heart.

oo oo oo

DIANE DI PRIMA

from: Nativity _____

> *The unbreakable fetters which*
> *bound down the Great Wolf Fenrir*
> *had been cunningly forged by Loki*
> *from these:*
> *The footfall of a cat,*
> *the roots of a rock*
> *the beard of a woman*
> *the breath of a fish*
> *the spittle of a bird. . . .*
> —*The Edda*

I.

Dark timbers of lost forests falling into my bed.
My hairs stirring, not asleep. Did they fetter me
with cat's paw, rock root, the beard
(o shame) of woman? They fettered me
w/ leather straps, on delivery table. I cd not
cry out. Forced gas mask over mouth,
slave. I cd not
turn head. Did they fetter me
w/ breath of a fish? These poison airs? I cd not
turn head, move hand, or leg
thus forced. They tore child from me. Whose?
What kind beast, near, breathing, what
royal hall or temple where I got this
slave flesh? Breath of a fish, the spittle
of a bird. So thin & slow. Seabirds cry at
full moon. But I. Cd not.
They fed thin soup & sour
reluctant milk. What prince
fathered this mite? Silence
sticky as cheese. Kind beasts around me: Women
who knew same outrage. Every child here
princeling, is shackled & numbered. We breathe
in our rags to keep each other warm.

TOI DERRICOTTE

from: *Natural Birth* _____

In my ninth month, I entered a maternity ward set up for
the care of unwed girls and women in Holy Cross Hospital.

HOLY CROSS HOSPITAL

couldn't stand to see these new young faces, these
children swollen as myself. my roommate, snotty,
bragging about how she didn't give a damn about the
kid and was going back to her boyfriend and be a
cheerleader in high school.   *could we ever "go back"?*
would our bodies be the same?   could we hide among the
childless?   she always reminded me of a lady at the bridge
club in her mother's shoes, playing her mother's hand.

i tried to get along, be silent, stay in my own corner.
i only had a month to go—too short to get to know them.
but being drawn to the room down the hall, the t.v. room
where, at night, we sat in our cuddly cotton robes and
fleece-lined slippers—like college freshmen, joking
about the nuns and laughing about due dates: jailbirds
waiting to be sprung . . .

one girl, taller and older, twenty-six or twenty-seven, kept
to herself, talked with a funny accent.   the pain on her face
seemed worse than ours . . .

and a lovely, gentle girl with flat small bones.   the
great round hump seemed to carry *her* around!   she never
said an unkind word to anyone, went to church every morning
with her rosary and prayed each night alone in her room.

she was seventeen, diabetic, fearful that she or the baby
or both would die in childbirth.   she wanted the baby, yet
knew that to keep it would be wrong.   but what if the child
did live?   what if she gave it up and could never have another?

i couldn't believe the fear, the knowledge she had of
death walking with her.   i never felt stronger, eating
right, doing my exercises. i was holding on to the core,

the center of strength; death seemed remote, i could not
imagine it walking in our midst, death in the midst of
all that blooming. . .

she went down two weeks late. induced. she had decided
to keep the baby. the night i went down, she had just
gone into labor so the girls had two of us to cheer about.
the next morning when i awoke, i went to see her. she
smiled from her hospital bed with tubes in her arms. it
had been a boy. her baby was dead in the womb for two
weeks. i remembered she had complained *no kicking*. we
had reassured her everything was fine.

meanwhile i worked in the laundry, folded the hospital
fresh sheets flat three hours a day.

                    . . .

i felt pretty, body wide and still in black beatnik
leotards, washed out at night. my shapely legs and
young body like iron.

i ate well, wanted lamaze (painless childbirth)—i
didn't need a husband or a trained doctor—i'd do it
myself, book propped open on the floor, puffing and
counting while all the sixteen-year-old unwed children
smiled like i was crazy.

one day i got a letter from my cousin, said:

> *don't give your baby up—*
> *you'll never be complete again*
> *you'll always worry where and how it is*

she knew! the people in my family knew! nobody died
of grief and shame!

i *would* keep the child. i was sturdy. would be a better
mother than my mother. i would still be a doctor,
study, finish school at night. when the time came, i
would not hurt like all those women who screamed and
took drugs. I would squat down and deliver just like the
peasants in the field, shift my baby to my back, and
continue . . .

when my water broke, when i saw that stain of pink blood
on the toilet paper and felt the first thing i could not
feel, had no control of, dripping down my leg, i heard
them singing mitch miller xmas songs and came from the
bathroom in my own pink song—down the long hall, down
the long moment when no one knew but me. it was time.

all the girls were cheering when i went downstairs. i was
the one who told them to be tough, to stop believing
in their mother's pain, that poison. our minds were
like telescopes looking through fear. it wouldn't hurt
like we'd been told. birth was beautiful if we believed
that it was beautiful and good!

—maternity—i had never seen inside those doors.
all night i pictured the girls up there, at first hanging
out of the windows, trying to get a glimpse of me ...
when the pain was worst, i thought of their sleeping faces,
like the shining faces of children in the nursery. i held
onto that image of innocence like one light in the darkness.

. . .

MATERNITY

when they checked me in, i was thinking: *this is going to be
a snap*! but at the same time, everything looked so different!
this was another world, ordered and white. the night moved
by on wheels.

suddenly the newness of the bed, the room, the quiet,
the hospital gown they put me in, the sheets rolled up
hard and starched and white and everything white except the
clock on the wall in red and black and the nurse's back as
she moved out of the room without speaking, everything
conspired to make me feel afraid.

how long, how much will i suffer?

the night looked in from bottomless windows.

going to the bathroom.   worse than cramps.   can't stop
going to the bathroom.   shaking my head over the toilet.
just sit.   sit on the toilet.   don't move.   just shake
your head.   try to go so hard.   maybe it will go away.
just try.   press real hard.   *it hurts   i can't help it   oh
it hurts so bad!*

lie on the bed and can't breathe right.   go to sleep and
wake up in the middle of a wave, too late ...

what time is it, i can't keep track of time ...

fall asleep.   two minutes.   can't stand the pain.   have
to go to the bathroom.   feels so ugly pressing down there,
shame, shame!   have to go to the bathroom all the time.
shake my head.   can't believe it hurts like this and
getting worse.

lie back in bed, just breathe.   just relax.   watch the
clock.   one minute goes so slow.   seems like 10:29, the
clock is stuck there, stuck on pain ...

nurse comes in, asks me if i want a shot.   *no i don't want a
shot.   i want this to be easy.   please god make it easy, i said it
would be easy.   no i don't want a shot don't want to give up
yet, i want it to be beautiful like it's supposed to be if i just
breathe right, can't give up they want me to give up i won't
give up*   (the minutes stuck around the clock),   *please
nobody see me* (the nurse says the social worker wants to
see me ... and the social worker is pregnant!)   *god don't
let her see.   i told her to have lamaze like me told her it was
easy and not to be afraid.   don't let her see how hard don't
let her be afraid like i am now.   never again, never have a
baby, never believe that this is beautiful or good
i'm rolling in the dark   the clock is stuck   the big black clock
is stuck.   inside i'm quiet outside i roll and can't
stop it getting worse, can't stop   it's getting worse—it can't
get worse!   how could a body hold such pain?   how could
such pain be here and how and what did i do?   i want to
scream   i can't.   my mouth is stopped   my mouth is dry—
so dry   god let me out of this hell   i did my exercises loved
my baby did everything i could, you promised if i was good*

you promised if i was clean and pure and beautiful, if i was
humble like a child and loved them all the little children
(so far to the bathroom, so cold in the night loving my baby,
so far, so cold, so long) *and no one to come and save me*
from this pain i cannot stop oh god no one to save me....

. . .

the nurse says she'll give me a shot.   still wants to
give me a shot.   *but i don't want a shot.   i've tried so hard*
all night to stay awake and fight and breathe, and now it's
8:00 and might go on like this forever   i want to be awake
and see my baby, want to see him crown, the head immense
as sun and bright with blood crack over the bowl of earth   i
want to feel the womb of god close over me, and want to,
more than anything, feel joy and love and welcome him   god
help this man be born into this world   help   his mother wants
to share this moment with his beauty   wants to hold on to
the pain a second more and feel him crown inside me   majesty
and might   no more than being humble will allow a broken
woman, let me be awake and push him into light . . .

it's light outside   it's light   i can see it in the mirror
day is coming   night is passing   i am so far in myself
i can't see out   can't say no to anything floating on my
pain . . .

doctor comes in to feel the head.   keeps coming in,
making me hurt, sticking his whole hand up my asshole.
and it hurts like sticking a wooden ax handle up my cunt
and grinding it inside me, hot cigars burning ax handles
and i can't move i'm in such pain, can't move away from
him raping me each time sticking his whole gloved hand
up my wounded cunt.

. . .

he wants me to roll and beg like a dog, *please doctor*
please don't hurt me   do anything   do anything you
say   but help me   help me not to feel such pain   but i don't
beg him.   i don't beg him because i hate him.   i keep

my pain locked up inside.   he'll never know how much
he hurts, i'll never let him know.

my heart is frozen like a calf.   on ice.   my heart is
empty meat.   my heart, my love is frozen.   i will never
love again.

TRANSITION

the meat rolls up and moans on the damp table.
my body is a piece of cotton over another
woman's body.   some other woman, all muscle and nerve, is
tearing apart and opening under me.

i move with her like skin, not able to do anything else,
i am just watching her, not able to believe what her
body can do, what it *will* do, to get this thing accomplished.

this muscle of a lady, this crazy ocean in my teacup.
she moves the pillars of the sky.   i am stretched into
fragments, tissue paper thin.   the light shines through
to her goatness, her blood-thick heart that thuds like
one drum in the universe emptying its stars.

she is
that heart
larger
than my life
stuffed
in
me
like sausage
black sky
bird
pecking
at the bloody
ligament

trying
to get
in, get
out
i am

holding out with
everything i
have
holding out
the evil thing

when i see there is
no answer
to the screamed
word
GOD
nothing i can do,
no use,
i have to let her in,
open the door,
put down the mat
welcome her
as if she
might be the
called for death,
the final
abstraction.

she comes
like a tunnel
fast
coming into
blackness
with my headlights
off

            you can push . . .

i hung there, still hurting, not knowing what to do.
if you push too early, it hurts more.   i called the
doctor back again.   *are you sure i can push?   are you sure?*

i couldn't believe that pain was over, that the punishment was enough, that the wave, the huge blue mind i
was living inside, was receding.   i had forgotten there
ever was a life without pain, a moment when pain wasn't
absolute as air.

why weren't the nurses and doctors rushing toward me?
why weren't they wrapping me in white? white for respect,
white for triumph, white for the white light i was being
accepted into after death? why was it so simple as saying
you can push? why were they walking away from me into
other rooms as if this were not the end the beginning of
something which the world should watch?

i felt something pulling me inside, a soft call, but i
could feel her power. something inside me i could go
with, wide and deep and wonderful. the more i gave
to her, the more she answered me. i held this conversation
in myself like a love that never stops. i pushed toward
her, she came toward me, gently, softly, sucking like a
wave. i pushed deeper and she swelled wider, darker when
she saw i wasn't afraid. then i saw the darker glory
of her under me.

why wasn't the room bursting with lilies? why was
everything the same with them moving so slowly as if
they were drugged? why were they acting the same when,
suddenly, everything had changed?

we were through with pain, would never suffer in our
lives again. put pain down like a rag, unzipper skin,
step out of our dead bodies, and leave them on the
floor. glorious spirits were rising, blanched with
light, like thirsty women shining with their thirst.

oo oo oo

LAURIE COLWIN

from: Another Marvelous Thing _____

Billy lay on a gurney, waiting to be rolled down the hall. Grey, wearing hospital scrubs, stood beside her holding her hand. She had been prepped and given an epidural anesthetic, and she could no longer feel her legs.

"Look at me," she said to Grey. "I'm a mass of tubes. I'm a miracle of modern science." She put his hand over her eyes.

Grey squatted down to put his head near hers. He looked expectant, exhausted, and worried, but when he saw her scanning his face he smiled.

"It's going to be swell," Grey said. "We'll find out if it's little William or little Ella."

Billy's heart was pounding but she thought she ought to say something to keep her side up. She said, "I knew we never should have had sexual intercourse." Grey gripped her hand tight and smiled. Eva laughed. "Don't you guys leave me," Billy said.

Billy was wheeled down the hall by an orderly. Grey held one hand, Eva held the other. Then they left her to scrub.

She was taken to a large, pale green room. Paint was peeling on the ceiling in the corner. An enormous lamp hung over her head. The anesthetist appeared and tapped her feet.

"Can you feel this?" he said.

"It doesn't feel like feeling," Billy said. She was trying to keep her breathing steady.

"Excellent," he said.

Then Jordan appeared at her feet, and Grey stood by her head.

Eva bent down. "I know you'll hate this, but I have to tape your hands down, and I have to put this oxygen mask over your face. It comes off as soon as the baby's born, and it's good for you and the baby."

Billy took a deep breath. The room was very hot. A screen was placed over her chest.

"It's so you can't see," said Eva. "Here's the mask. I know it'll freak you out, but just breathe nice and easy. Believe me, this is going to be fast."

Billy's arms were taped, her legs were numb, and a clear plastic mask was placed over her nose and mouth. She was so frightened she wanted to cry out, but it was impossible. Instead she breathed as Katherine Walden had taught her to. Every time a wave of panic rose, she

116

breathed it down. Grey held her hand. His face was blank and his glasses were fogged. His hair was covered by a green cap and his brow was wet. There was nothing she could do for him, except squeeze his hand.

"Now, Billy," said Jordan Bell, "you'll feel something cold on your stomach. I'm painting you with Betadine. All right, here we go."

Billy felt something like dull tugging. She heard the sound of foamy water. Then she felt the baby being slipped from her. She turned to Grey. His glasses had unfogged and his eyes were round as quarters. She heard a high, angry scream.

"Here's your baby," said Jordan Bell. "It's a beautiful, healthy boy."

Eva lifted the mask off Billy's face.

"He's perfectly healthy," Eva said. "Listen to those lungs." She took the baby to be weighed and tested. Then she came back to Billy. "He's perfect but he's little—just under five pounds. We have to take him upstairs to the preemie nursery. It's policy when they're not five pounds."

"Give him to me," Billy said. She tried to free her hands but they were securely taped.

"I'll bring him to you," Eva said. "But he can't stay down here. He's too small. It's for the baby's safety, I promise you. Look, here he is."

The baby was held against her forehead. The moment he came near her he stopped shrieking. He was mottled and wet.

"Please let me have him," Billy said.

"He'll be fine," Eva said. They then took him away.

oo oo oo

NICOLE BROSSARD

from: *Journal intime* _____

      The water, when the waters break and I won't know anything about it, lying on an operating table, for, Caesar, open yourself, wade through our bellies during caesarians and the mothers sleep an exemplary sleep. Anesthetized. The mothers are hot, cold, they tremble, revive, fling themselves about and bawl in hospitals. The mothers sign a great x on their children's eyes, sign the end of the eternal return when they leave the hospital or they leave reality or they leave with a great x on their bellies. Yes the mothers have all the assets and all the charms for the x's that dance in their eyes, the mothers have obligations, appointments, the mothers have the breath of the deepest silence. The mothers suddenly want the sea and the salt just as the amazons must, gazing at the sea, have tasted the salt of their sister lovers, as a reality, the mothers become grave and they begin gravitating around their center of gravity and then they float, aerial, the mothers who invent humanity by inventing their daughters in their image and in the haziness of that image, the mothers invent their lives like tigresses, the mothers light up the eyes of she-wolves in the most distant patriarchal steppe and the she-wolves become women in the curve of humanity's lens. Then once this is done, the mothers say they don't have time to keep up their journals. And then we hear only their voices and their voices are never altogether their voices. These are voices that travel out to the horizon like little clouds. And life is organized despite their loving phrases and life scratches out their sobs.

APRIL 24, 1974.

I see you, I look at you. *Intensely* is only a word. This is a lightning bolt, body and soul for my whole life. Lightning, light, energy. Yours, life to come. You are my daughter a day reality and fiction crossed. You are the one called The Nasturtium and through you the world is an April day luminous in your black hair. My sweetly shaggy one, I dreamed that when you were born you already knew how to talk.

—translated by Lydia Davis

ALICE HOFFMAN

from: *Fortune's Daughter* _____

The night grew so cold that when it began to rain the drops froze the moment they hit the sidewalk. There were hundreds of accidents: cars and buses skidded on the icy avenues, lights in hotel rooms flickered as generators came to a halt, pipes froze and then burst, and every frail tree in the city was hidden beneath a shower of ice. Up in her room, Lila was surrounded by black fire. She might have slipped into the darkness forever if her cousin Ann hadn't arrived a little after midnight. The bedroom door opened slowly, and the scraping of wood against wood sounded like the flapping of some huge bird's wings. Lila gasped when the sudden light from the hallway filled her room. For one calm moment Lila wondered if she had imagined the pain, and she watched as her cousin took off her gray wool coat and her leather boots. Before the bedroom door was closed Lila had enough time to look out and see her mother peer into the bedroom. At least, Lila thought it was her mother—she wore her mother's clothes, and was her mother's shape and size. But if it really had been her mother, wouldn't she have run into the room and thrown her arms around her daughter and tried to save her? Lila blinked and strained to see, but the figure in the hallway just grew shadowier, and when Lila's cousin walked toward the door she blocked the light, and then there weren't even any shadows. There was nothing at all.

When the door closed the sound echoed. Lila could actually feel the sound somewhere beneath her skin. Immediately the room was airless; the heat in the radiator poured out until it was impossible to breathe. That was when Lila knew she couldn't have this baby.

"I'm sorry," she told her cousin. "They made you come here for nothing. I've changed my mind. I'm not going through with this."

Ann had been a nurse for eleven years—long enough to know she had better not tell Lila that every woman in hard labor had made the exact same pronouncement.

"I can't do this!" Lila screamed.

Every neighbor on the floor above could hear her now for all she cared. Her contractions had been coming two minutes apart for some time, but now something changed. She could no longer tell the difference between one contraction and the next; the pain began to run together in a single line of fire. As each contraction rose to its highest peak, hot liquid poured out between Lila's legs. She couldn't sit, or lie down—she couldn't stand. Ann helped her onto the bed and examined her. By the time she was through, Lila was so wet that the sheets beneath her were soaked.

"Give me something," she begged. "Give me a shot. Put me out. Do anything."

The pain owned her now; it owned the earth and the air and at its center was an inferno. She was in the darkest time before birth, transition, and even though she didn't know its name, Lila knew, all of a sudden, that she could not go back. There was nothing to go back to, there was only this pain—and it was stronger than she was. It was swallowing her alive.

She wanted Hannie, that was all there was to it. In the past few weeks she had considered going to see her a hundred times, but a hundred times her pride got in the way, and now it was too late. She tried to imagine the stiff black skirts, and the clucking sound Hannie made in the back of her throat, and couldn't. There was nothing but this room, and inside the room there was only pain. And even if Hannie had been right beside her, Lila would still have been alone. That was the unbearable part of this pain—no one could accompany you, no one could share it, and the absolute loneliness of it was nearly enough to drive you mad.

Ann went to the bathroom to dampen some washcloths, and when she came back she found Lila standing by the window, looking out. The sidewalk was three stories down, and from this distance the ice that had formed on the cement seemed as cool and delicious as a deep, blue bay in Maine. Ann ran and turned her away from the window. It did no good to think of an escape, or even to wish for one. This was the center of it, and all you had to do was stand your ground—you could not even think about giving up.

When she saw the damp washcloths, Lila grabbed one out of her cousin's hand and sucked out the water. She was dying of thirst. She would have given anything for a piece of ice, a lemonade, a cool place where she could drift into a deep and dreamless sleep.

"Please," Lila said to her cousin.

"Just remember," Ann said, "I'm not going to leave you. I'm going to stay right here with you till the end."

"You can't leave me!" Lila cried, terrified and misunderstanding.

"I won't," Ann told her. "I'm right here."

Lila threw her arms around Ann's neck. She had never wanted to be closer to anyone. Again and again she whispered "please," but she knew there was no one who could save her. And then something let loose inside Lila, and it was simply beyond her powers to hold it back. She felt a terrible urge to push this thing inside of her out, and when

Ann told her she couldn't push yet, she started to cry. Ann showed her how to pant—it was a trick to fool her body into believing it was breathing that she must concentrate on—but even then Lila's tears ran into the back of her throat and nearly made her choke. Nothing was working, she couldn't even pant; she took in more and more air until she started to hyperventilate. Ann began to breathe along with her, and eventually Lila was able to slow her panting to match her cousin's. Lila stared into Ann's eyes and the room fell away from her; the city no longer existed. She fell deeper into those eyes—they were the universe, filled with energy and unbelievable light. Lila heard a voice tell her to get back onto the bed. She didn't feel herself move, and yet there she was, on those damp white sheets with her legs pulled up.

"It's time," Lila heard someone say to her. "Now you can push."

For a moment everything was clear. Lila recognized the ceiling in her bedroom, and the face of her cousin who was a hospital nurse. It seemed that a serious mistake had been made. This could not possibly be happening to her.

It was day now, but the air was so cold that the dawn was blue. Lila sat up in bed; she leaned back against the pillows and pulled her legs up as far as they could go. She pushed for the first time, and when she did she was horrified to hear her own voice. Surely, a sound like that would tear a throat apart. She pushed again, and again, but after more than an hour there was still the same enormous pressure. The only difference was now Lila was so exhausted that she couldn't even scream. All she wanted was for this horrible burning thing inside her to come out. She found herself thinking the same odd phrase over and over. It's only your body, she told herself. It was her flesh that had betrayed her, her blood that was on fire. The solution was simple and took only an instant. As her cousin leaned over her and wiped her face with a washcloth, as dawn reflected through windows all over the city, Lila left her body behind.

Her spirit leapt up into the pure white air. The utter joy of such a leap was almost too much for her. Lila rose upward, guided by a perfect beam of light. Below her, she could see her body propped up on two pillows, she could see that her eyes were closed, and that she held her breath as she pushed down with all the strength she had left. But how could she be concerned with a body that twisted and groaned, something that was so far away. Up here, in this strange new atmosphere, everything was silent. The air was so cold it crystallized, and each time Lila opened her mouth to breathe it quenched her thirst. There was the scent of something much sweeter than roses, and Lila wasn't the least bit surprised to find that her spirit had taken the shape of a bird. What else but a blackbird could swoop so gracefully above a room of pain?

"So now you're free," someone was saying to Lila. "Now you know that absolute freedom of leaving your body behind."

"It was so easy to do," Lila said. "How could anything be this easy?"

Far below her, Lila could hear her cousin ask who on earth she was talking to. But Lila didn't bother to answer. Any moment she might have to return to her body, each second was too precious to waste. The blue dawn was nothing compared to the white light that Lila had discovered. And when the time came for her to return to her body, Lila felt such a terrible sorrow that for an instant she thought she might choose not to return at all. She was floating just above herself, still undecided, when she suddenly found herself moved by the struggle beneath her. Her body's shallow breathing and the beat of her own heart filled Lila with pity; with one tender motion she slipped back inside her own flesh.

This time when she pushed, something hard moved so that it was nearly out. Lila reached her hands between her legs and felt the soft hair on the very top of the baby's head.

"Oh, my God," Lila said.

"The next time you push you may feel as if you'll explode," Ann said. "You may feel like you're burning."

But Lila had already been a spear of flame; she could dance on red coals now and not feel a thing. She bore down harder, and suddenly the baby's head was free. Lila panted again to stop the urge to push while Ann untangled the umbilical cord from around the neck, and then, with the next push, the entire body slipped out in a rush.

Blood poured from Lila, but she felt strangely renewed. She leaned her elbows on the pillows and lifted herself up so that she could watch as Ann cleaned off the baby and wrapped it in a white towel.

"Is it all right?" she whispered.

"It's perfect," Ann told her. "And it's a girl."

Lila's father had come home from a night spent out on the stairway, where it was so cold it could freeze your soul. He and his wife sat on the couch in the living room, rocking back and forth as if in mourning. Behind the closed bedroom door, Ann placed the baby in a dresser drawer on a bed of flannel nightgowns. It wasn't until after she had delivered the placenta that she told Lila that her parents had already had her contact a doctor who arranged private adoptions.

"But I have to have your approval," Ann told Lila.

Lila leaned her head back on the pillows and closed her eyes while Ann lifted her legs and put down a clean sheet.

"You have to tell me," Ann said. "What do you want to do about this child?"

What amazed Lila was how fast it was over, how far outside herself she had gone and how quickly she had returned. Already, the pain she'd felt seemed to belong to someone else. How strange that now she didn't want it to fade—she wanted to grab on to the pain and claim it for her own.

"I'll be honest with you," Ann said. "I don't really see how you can keep this baby. If you do, your parents won't let you stay here. Is it fair to keep her, when you can't even take care of yourself?"

Even though the steam heat in the radiator made a gurgling noise, and buses trapped in the ice strained their engines, Lila swore she could hear her baby breathing as it slept in the dresser drawer. It was at that moment that her heart broke in two: she knew she could not keep this child.

"I want to see her," Lila said.

"Take my advice," Ann told her. "If you plan to give her up, don't see her. Let me just take her away."

"I know what I want," Lila said. "Let me see her."

As soon as her daughter was brought to her and she held her in her arms, Lila knew her cousin was right. But instead of turning her away, Lila held the baby even tighter. Her skin was as soft as apricots, her eyes were the color of an October sky. Lila could have held her forever. She begged for time to stop, for clocks to break, for every star to remain fixed. But none of that happened. Up on the fourth floor the neighbors ran the water in the bathroom, in the hallway outside the apartment there was the scent of coffee.

When Lila gave her daughter up to her cousin's outstretched arms, the room grew darker, as if she had given away a star. The dresser drawer where her baby had slept was still open, and it would be days before Lila would be able to close it again. But now, as her child was taken out into the coldest winter morning ever recorded in the city, wrapped in nothing but a white towel, Lila did manage to get one last look, and for the first time she knew the loss she would feel from that day onward, every morning and every night, for the rest of her life.

oo oo oo

ERICA JONG

On the First Night _____

On the first night
of the full moon,
the primeval sack of ocean
broke,
& I gave birth to you
little woman,
little carrot top,
little turned-up nose,
pushing you out of myself
as my mother
pushed
me out of herself,
as her mother did,
& her mother's mother before her,
all of us born
of woman.

I am the second daughter
of a second daughter
of a second daughter,
but you shall be the first.
You shall see the phrase
"second sex"
only in puzzlement,
wondering how anyone,
except a madman,
could call you "second"
when you are so splendidly
first,
conferring even on your mother
firstness, vastness, fullness
as the moon at its fullest
lights up the sky.
Now the moon is full again
& you are four weeks old.
Little lion, lioness,
yowling for my breasts,
growling at the moon,

how I love your lustiness,
your red face demanding,
your hungry mouth howling,
your screams, your cries
which all spell life
in large letters
the color of blood.

You are born a woman
for the sheer glory of it,
little redhead, beautiful screamer.
You are no second sex,
but the first of the first;
& when the moon's phases
fill out the cycle
of your life,
you will crow
for the joy
of being a woman,
telling the pallid moon
to go drown herself
in the blue ocean,
& glorying, glorying, glorying
in the rosy wonder
of your sunshining wondrous
self.

oo oo oo

LAURA CHESTER

from: *The Stone Baby* _____

"Did you know that the uterus is the strongest muscle in the human body," Martine announced. She always had these facts. "And that includes the biggest bicep of the strongest man on earth."

Julia smiled. She liked the idea, but she didn't want to talk. It had started to rain, and a light effervescence pumped the air—cool, damp, exhilerating.

As soon as they reached the deserted lobby of the hospital, Julia's stomach hit stop. She rushed toward the bathroom down the corridor, banged in and let it go, heave after heave. She probably shouldn't have eaten.

"You'll feel so much better now," Martine encouraged, but Julia felt overwhelmed.

The nurse in charge of Labor & Delivery was phoning for the alternative birth assistant. She arrived within minutes. Everything was clicking—Dr. Chou was on call, the rain—a good sign, the quiet evening on the floor, the availability of the room. Martine was right beside her, concerned, as present as her own body, and they were moving together in this. Julia tried not to think about Philip, how he should have been there too. She jerked herself back from that thought with the start of the next contraction. She needed the Lamaze breathing now. Martine held up 2,3, or 4 fingers, for a rhythm of pant-pant-blow. The labor was getting so strong, and Julia felt that she might get weepy. Thank God Martine was with her. How could she do this, like Martine had, eighteen years ago, alone?

The nurse said that she was already six centimeters dilated, and Julia was beginning to shift into that other world of intense concentration, the rugged, strained part of the climb, no switch-backs now, transition.

Dr. Chou appeared and the room buzzed with extra activity. They got the lighting right, and now her moans were getting higher, harder to keep down in the low zone. Between contractions, Julia stripped off her clothes. She didn't want anything on, so hot, and not embarrassed. For now she got down to work, *down*. It was all so fast. With every extreme contraction, she began to throw her head about, almost frantic.

"Look at the rose," Martine reminded, "look into the opening rose." She turned the flower on the bedside table, and Julia tried to focus, but she only wanted to look out, far far away, absenting herself from her body. She looked to Dr. Chou, and felt like her eyes were pleading, helplessly pleading with him to help. It hurt *it hurt* It Hurt IT HURT, beyond bearable, beyond a sane amount of pain, and when Dr. Chou examined her, it felt like human torture. "Philip," she cried, "Where are you!" She suddenly felt defeated, and Martine appeared confused.

"If you feel like pushing now, you can push," Dr. Chou said calmly, but that seemed next to impossible. They had just arrived. Could it happen so fast? It never had before.

"Pretty soon you're going to have your baby," the nurse whispered, wiping her forehead with a cool washcloth. Julia took it in her hands. She wanted cool! clean! hands! But she didn't feel the urge to push. Why not?

"I feel no urge," she protested.

"You're definitely ten centimeters," the doctor said, with his hand inside her, and Julia's waters burst, spraying his glasses and hospital gown. He was laughing. They were all laughing, everyone but Julia, who wanted them all to shut up! She was so serious, engaged, in the middle of a fierce contraction.

And so she began to push, not with the urge so much as from memory, from training. She knew how to grab the outside of her knees, and press down with a chest of breath, pushing with all her upper muscles. It did seem to help control the contractions, pushing down on their incredible intensity with her own. As soon as the contraction was over, she wanted a tiny ice chip, and Martine was there to serve her, reheating washcloths for her perineum, cold washcloths for her face and hands. She only had a minute to get ready for the next bout. Her hair seemed drenched. She was sweaty and slippery. "And I never even perspire," she laughed, weakly, but then—OH! She pushed *she pushed* She Pushed SHE PUSHED with all her might, and out came, shit. She lay her head back on the pillows, while they wiped it up and whisked it away, making nothing of it.

"Nothing's happening," she wailed.

But Martine said, "Just push that baby down and out. A little further, a little past the place where it was before." With Martine's encouragement, and the nurse's optimism, Dr. Chou's kind face, things progressed—"You're doing well! That's great, Julia. Embrace the pain, reach out to it. *Now* you're really getting somewhere."

She had no idea of how much time was passing, adrift in another world, thrown into it, laid back from it, though sometimes she felt lost in it, rather than making the best of each contraction, not bearing down thoroughly enough, missing the rhythm. Then she began to think that they were lying. They were simply being nice, at her expense. Encouragement was a useless token. The head *wasn't* descending. She couldn't believe it when Dr. Chou said that the head was through the cervix, and the body was entering the birth canal. It didn't feel that way at all.

But what was this? They wanted her up? They wanted her up on her feet and off to the bathroom. Sitting on the toilet, they said, would give her the advantage of gravity, help get that baby down. Their hands supported her on all sides, as she walked, bending and shuffling forward, and then squatting, she pulled at the back of Martine's blue jeans, until she thought she would rip the pockets off.

"You have to push through the pain, push *through* it," Martine coached, and Julia felt it descend. The nurse was pressing on Martine to support the weight, the mightiness of it. Yes, this was helping. Back she was maneuvered to bed, in a near weepy, out-of-it state, not sure if she could keep this up much longer.

Then they held a mirror down for Julia to see how her perineum was changing, but she only saw a mess of blood, and wanted it wiped away. Now she could see she was flattening out, and the nurse instructed her to place her fingers inside and touch the baby's head. Two inches inside she could feel a jellied mass that was her baby's head! She realized that this little person was close, so very close. She really felt that she was in the hands of God, and God's force was moving through her, and this seemed neither bad nor good, just a fact, and even though she thought—'This is agony,' the pain almost had an exquisite quality.

The nurse wanted her to keep her fingers inside with the next push to feel the progress.

"Why don't you speak to the baby," Martine said. These would be the last few moments that her baby would be living inside her.

Suddenly everyone seemed to be getting excited. Dr. Chou was putting on his gloves. They just had to get it down under that pubic bone, down and up and out and here. She was becoming more determined now. Down, down, come on baby, the gut crusher of will power. Every muscle in her neck, face, jaw, shoulders, arms, back and abdomen was straining, pushing, out and under and *down*. "Just a couple more pushes and you'll have your baby," the nurse's tone brought Julia back again to the bigger reality, that this wasn't just a fight against her own body, but a process that involved another human being, who was working too and being worked. And yet it seemed to go on. Martine held up the mirror, and yes, she thought she could see the littlest part of head crowning, and then a good fifty-cent-size piece of brown wet hair, and that made her push even harder, though she was filling up past the full point, stretching now past all possible limits, burning, and she thought, cool, *cool*, to no avail, for it felt like a raw hot split, stretching with nowhere to go. But then, after that contraction, the head slid back in a ways.

"That's good, Julia," the doctor said. "Just one more push like that one and you've got it." She believed him, and she put all her strength behind it.

Martine felt like a witness on some other level, pouring heart and energy into these last few moments—the anticipation, the struggle with the strain of it, the immensity, awesome, and it was almost as if huge music were on the way and she could hear it approaching, getting closer and closer, and stronger and more powerful, mounting up to overwhelm them all, and then, as if in a movie, "I've got to do a little snip here now," the instant decision, the ready move, when he saw that she wasn't going to give, and with that one easy snip he reached in for the chin, she was howling *ugh*, and crying *oh*, and she thought she'd be ripped apart, and Martine saw the head coming out as Julia's flesh tore like a split open grapefruit, and the head, which had appeared to be small, became gigantic. They pushed Julia over on her side, to turn the shoulders and then suddenly gush, so primitive, this huge chubby person was between her legs, humped up in a ball and she only felt what —immediate relief.

It was squirming in the doctor's hands, and Julia asked, "What is it?"

Somebody said, "I think it's a girl. Yes, it looks like a nice big baby girl."

Julia looked to the child and cried, she just started to bawl, "A girl? A *girl*! I can't believe it. Oh my God, a baby girl." And then Martine was crying too, and hugging her hard, and then Julia lay back, all quivering and high on the gut swinging chorus of altitude awe, booming and soaring, a tangible heart clap, sweet purse of the body rising straight up the spine, and it felt like the lid of the entire room, the entire building, was blown right off with this arrival, and there was such gratitude too, as Julia took that baby on her belly, touching her real live skin, her head, and leaning forward, her tears fell upon the child and she smoothed that little back, as the nurse began working on her. She had to gently massage Julia's uterus, while Julia continued to stroke the baby there on her chest, and out came the placenta easily, and then Dr. Chou began to sew, but nothing could distract Julia from this wonderful being, fresh from another world.

oo oo oo

BERNADETTE MAYER

from: *The Desires of Mothers to Please Others in Letters* _____

Everybody calls wondering where the baby is but the worst thing is
  nobody writes to make the days less empty, no letters means
  fear of dying
The overwhelming advent of baby on the business of scenes next week
  beginning again like one poor toe in an inch of hot bath
The midwife can reach into me and touch with two fingers the baby's
  true head
Still it has to come out, still saying so doesn't want it to
It's true writing is too exciting and lively and saintly
I'm another person, one child coughs the other's getting better
Absence of a tandem stroller, I've got cold feet, genuinely cold,
  it's zero
Remember the snapping air over white snow with blue smitten skies,
  twenty below one year
You could walk out and wonder, the air did not stir, could you breathe?
This is like leisure, I can't wait to hold the baby, no one around
First there was a cough and a cold, then we made this baby up, now
  it's near to full moon
Love of the light in the cold, the sumptuous ritual of birth,
  the spectacular cord
Heart beats faster so it must be a woman she said I mean a girl

      . . .

What do the contractions do, are they like *The Canterbury Tales?*
I heard the dog barking in this place arid of animals
More awakenings, days and nights, what was poetry
The help of the baby making a motion in the world you'd touch anyway
This cummerband of baby, this big old fat man, maybe jolly, this thing
  between my legs, there's a head there where my sex is
Past Santa Claus
The difference in days, so much the sweetest now
Drab light kept back from a heart like Cocteau mentions
I lean over the desk legs spread in the Gertrude-Stein skirt,
  a loose blouse like Emma Goldman who spoke at the
  laborlyceum

This hand, what will happen to this wrist or arm, I mean mine
Love of self, I am not in pain now, how could I ever be?
Baby lost or left, fallen, the drift of the packing of the shelf
Person gotten into being, again another one, now what we say is
    peace
        and now no more
          HEROIN, THE AGONIST-ANTAGONIST
A new cure for addiction, you pick things out from the world,
        I meant to say you choose them from the times
          "... fatter than a flat fur ..."
That's how it said the lynx makes you look
It's cold in here, what's it waiting for?
I guess it's cynical to be addicted to this cold weather
To pass the waiting time some words wind up in mind
So they say I am effaced but what will I do? Shall I withdraw
        from sight?

   . . .

Will you know, slight contraction later, how labor began, will you
        have been influenced and not by reason, telescoping memory
        like a mother does, she says when he was a baby then he was
        seven years old, he hit his head on that table over there
I sit still waiting before the pretty dawn like nearly everyone did,
        love is the same
Its form makes the speech, others have given birth, even tonight
The very seasons I can bother to picture the ultimate in nothing new
        comparing it to all
Which is why I am silent and cannot find an end to it, all this speaking
And photographing leaves, making love if it's o.k. to mention that
        Affecting babies, the children not the reason there is none
In some tribes and so on ...
So all life turns out to be the opposite of what half of everyone thought
& the reasons for continuing are the sources of stopping and silence
Not because of that but to add, all the stuff we thought was new is not
But I can't say that, I photographed the apparently empty field, I took
        its picture many times
Tonight you have a whiskey and I pride myself on drinking another beer
        at a time like this
When any moment I might be called on to lie back and climb a mountain
        for a while

   . . .

I lost it the days are awful, nights I still expect something
to happen, the woman smiled,
             I felt a great love for all women, women have memories
& many will look at me these days & feel so glad not to be me, it's
the end of the secret of women but not the end of the waiting for
what everyone's done already, there's the common knowledge of the
castor oil, the understanding of the overdue baby, the last baby, the
baby named or not named, the big pain in the ass, motion, dreams of
airplanes and people being pushed around in torn clothing, life full of
holes, maybe I know nothing, this time in the sense that if life were
less crazy I'd likely have less ignorance, dreams of the New Mexico
State Prison, the news of the day on the day of the birth, it probably
won't be the 6th now, the 7th or 8th, the phone rings incessantly
because I am bursting, it's hard, I mean like a stone with a letter of
the alphabet written on it, I don't know either whether to eat or
drink, the smell of the food is awful, taste of the metal beer, the
aluminum milk, the baby does something, I'm all both fucked up and
freaked out, I'm a wreck as they say, had one at 8:15, now I feel a
little sick, I get in some position and something starts happening but
then I move & it won't keep going, I'm impotent! My uterus must be
exhausted! I'm too old! The exuberance of all the false labors turns to
lethargy, defending against expectations, what a silly word, I still look
the same in the mirror, my face I mean my head does, where is the
midwife sleeping? in her bed? a funny hooting or creaking I hear once
in a while when it's quiet downstairs & at night when you're
sleeping, it must be the baby in the womb actually being already
outside me, children fighting all day, all day asking for little bits of
food they don't really want to eat, little single things, then those
things & foods not satisfying them they spit on the floor, throw the
stuff away and ask for more something, they say I need, I need,
should I get married and then destroy everything, should I take a
shower in Kiev or a bath? The mystical cop-out ambiguous
nineteenth-century ending of *Villette* Peggy said was a book wherein
you want to kick all the characters, babies sigh fear, no more babies,
never again, no more waiting, no sense of humor, why isn't my
mother or somebody waiting here with me, it'll never come back
again, it needs another woman, pity me Patty, phone rings, I think
it's someone calling to say the baby's born, it's over, thanks, thanks a
million, thanks for letting me know, she said my thoughts go with
you making me quake in my boots for fear I might be dying as well,
then she said of course it will all be fine & I know she never thinks
that's true she always thinks it will all be all wrong, fucked up,
upside down, fraught with complications, requiring surgery because

that's more interesting, hideous and unlucky, I stop & look around,
what am I saying, should I try a beer, will the beer lessen the chance
for contractions I aspire to tonight, I have them anyway, they go
nowhere, it does have to happen doesn't it, some squealing I hear it
again like a bannister squeaking like a person, to assure proper credit
please don't be like you are, I'm clumsy, I drop everything on the
floor, sometimes I even drop everything in the garbage by mistake,
when he saw me still encumbered he said oh you poor thing, today
we dropped all the cooked spaghetti in the sink and had to make it
new & the juice on the floor & I broke a dish and a cup by throwing
a bowl at them to make the children stop fighting, I'm getting mad
and I'm washing all the dishes though it's not my job, I'm exhausting
myself conserving energy then I see I'm much too tired to have the
baby now, I don't want the landlord to be here when the baby's born,
I want to have my baby alone with only Lewis and Carol, Suzanne
and Marie, Lewis dreamed a boy, the room was pale blue, they had
painted it for you, the supper & the day cold & dreary, I had to
teach my class

at the Bradford IGA
a woman smiled at me

we live in a bowl of small towns

> "It was like each person was a button on
> your coat"

now the foolish dog's come into the house
there is no privacy
it was sumptuous with another blue sky today
it must be on account of ovaries there are memories
the men could exist anytime
they can even freeze sperm

each country is black, the women are smiling & comparing journals,
the work of the past living in some other woman they might happen
to notice, they're ready for that, but the men, even the stoical silent
ice fishermen telling stories at the store don't have the feeling one
knows how the other must've felt so memory gets lost & is unknown
except that the man's dog barks again so the man remembers
someone must be coming & then of course there's a knocking and for
a second we're convinced we might be right

to bring forth issue

SHARON OLDS

The Language of the Brag _____

I have wanted excellence in the knife-throw,
I have wanted to use my exceptionally strong and
    accurate arms
and my straight posture and quick electric
    muscles
to achieve something at the center of a crowd,
the blade piercing the bark deep,
the shaft slowly and heavily vibrating like the
    cock.

I have wanted some epic use for my excellent
    body,
some heroism, some American achievement
beyond the ordinary for my extraordinary self,
magnetic and tensile, I have stood by the sandlot
and watched the boys play.

I have wanted courage, I have thought about fire
and the crossing of waterfalls, I have dragged
    around
my belly big with cowardice and safety,
my stool black with iron pills,
my huge breasts oozing mucus,
my legs swelling, my hands swelling,
my face swelling and darkening, my hair
falling out, my inner sex stabbed again and again
    with terrible pain
like a knife.
I have lain down.

I have lain down and sweated and shaken
and passed blood and feces and water and
slowly alone in the center of a circle I have
passed the new person out
and they have lifted the new person free of the
    act
and wiped the new person free of that
language of blood like praise all over the body.

I have done what you wanted to do, Walt
    Whitman,
Allen Ginsberg, I have done this thing,
I and the other women this exceptional
act with the exceptional heroic body,
this giving birth, this glistening verb,
and I am putting my proud American boast
right here with the others.

THE PAINFUL PARTS

oo oo oo

CHRISTINE SCHUTT

Sisters _____

Last summer my younger sister Trimble and her husband Peter left the city for a two-story shuttered house in Connecticut with room to spare for children, if they should be lucky enough to have children. My sister has problems: she is missing some parts and what is there—enough—doesn't quite work as it should, so that now she sees her body as something apart, a shadow, stumped or lengthening depending on the date with one high-noon dissolve when, for a short while, she is all of a piece and the air is moted with possibility. On these days, she walks on tiptoe, squinting into the bright light of the future with all the earnest, hopeful purpose she once displayed when at age sixteen she raised her verbal score some two hundred points. On these days, when she asks me, "And the boys? How are the boys?" I am sad. She has always been such a good girl; I want to tell her *that* counts for something.

Instead, when my sister talks to me our eyes don't meet; every line of hers trails into ellipses, and I'm left feeling dumb and out of it. She tells me about the drugs she's taking, then stops, and when I say, "Go on," she answers from a distance, "Not much more to tell." I want to touch her but the remembered sensation of the fleshy pouch beneath her arms whenever I took hold of her to guide her out of my room—"off limits to punks"—needles me. Since my divorce, I've become the younger sister, and Trimble is off limits to me.

I sit in her new kitchen and watch her roll the dough for the cookies we've come to help decorate, the cookies my grandmother, and after her, I, used to make. My youngest son sorts through the cutters—the roosters, reindeers, santas, bells—amazed at newfound treasure. "I don't remember these," he says.

"I do," my older boy brags. "This one is mine, isn't it, Mom?"

And even though none of the cutters is tagged, I say, "Yes," because I'm grateful for any reminders of a life before, when I baked, had dinners, and spent the early hours of the morning with my young husband, cleaning up after the guests, recalling talk while chinging the crystal clean: young, comfortable, happier than we knew. I want to tell my sister what I'm feeling, but she's told me she hates the man, he was a shit, I should forget him.

She slaps her hands and clouds of flour rain on the boys. "Now your hair is as gray as mine," she says. "Didn't you tell me my hair was getting so white?" She pokes at Sean and moves to pull Brendon to her, Brendon, who at ten has already grown past her shoulder. Not that she's small; he's big. "Brendon," she croons and is about to launch into how she knew him when he seizes on another cutter and holds up the naked lady.

"Awesome!" he shouts.

"Titties," Sean joins in.

"Bazooms, and," Brendon points at vacant space.

"Guys," Trimble is blushing for them.

I pull Sean onto my lap. "Cool it," I say, nod firmly at Brendon. "Why don't you go draw? We brought all that paper with us. Do something constructive. The cookies won't be ready to decorate for a while."

Trimble ruffles the flour out of their hair as they pass by. "Draw me a picture," she says. "Draw me a picture of my house." She follows them into the den. "Draw a picture of the house for Peter and me."

Every weekend Trimble and her husband make improvements on their house. The den is one such change; the room was once a garage. Always off the kitchen, on a lower level of land, it is now a quiet strip of beach, cool and green with white wall-to-wall carpet. The boys like to roll from one end to another. I feel like a kid in there, too.

Trimble likes to tell people that when she was growing up I was mean to her. She was too young to know how I used to make her laugh, playing with her boingy curls. After our parents' divorce, when we moved in with Nana, we grew apart because Trimble wanted everyone back together again, and I knew that wouldn't happen. Trimble remembers a fight we had then, and how she slept in a bathtub on a vacation we took with Nana. I have to remind her, "That was the night you said Mother should live with us. And I said you were crazy. I said she was a black blot in our lives."

"I remember," Trimble says in her haunted-house voice. "I was scared. I thought of ink on paper."

Other times, moments when Nana captioned, "You won't see this again, girls," we drew together in amazement at our lives. Assassinations, scandals: the lidless public eye fossilized events at a glance. On the night of the 1968 Democratic Convention, I took Trimble for a drive to listen to the radio reports of riots and to wonder at the quiet along the county roads, the sequined light, the soft sleep two hours north of Chicago. We pulled over onto the shoulder of Highway 83 and under a junction light slow jitter-bugged to an old Everly Brothers song: *Bye, bye love; bye, bye happiness.* Recalling this night, Trimble always says, "For once you weren't stoned and drawling nonsense."

The first batch of cookies burns. Too thin and set too close together, the edges are black and blurred. Trimble scoops the shapeless cookies onto paper towels and calls out to the boys, "First batch ready for testing." They swarm over the fragrant mound, picking up clusters and bells stuck together. We start to cut the dough thicker, grease the sheets good. Sean keeps watch of things in the oven. When I smile at him, he smiles back: good little boy with no front teeth and greasy chin buttery-yellow.

"Earth to Trimble!" he calls because she says it to him all the time, and she's so tickled by his joke, she hugs him and fusses until he squirms away. "Aunt Trimble! The cookies!"

"The cookies?" she pretends surprise.

Brendon nudges. "I dib the tree."

The kitchen smells of vanilla, and the goofy Siamese is snuffing the corners and batting loose silver candies over the floor. Flour settles on the rack of dishes like a dusting of snow. The counters are sticky. I am happy in all this confusion and sponge clean some space, mumbling about how we haven't even begun to frost yet! when I'm thinking maybe next month it will happen, and then next year there will be a baby upstairs, and we will buy special cutters—a different teddy, maybe a rocking horse—and scenes of how things will be roll giddy and bright as colored sugar pellets the cat's got into, when there's a sudden howl from Sean, and the hot sheet he's grabbed clatters to the floor.

Sean is crying, and everyone is screaming, Ice! Ice!

"Put his hand in cold water, Trimble," I say, filling up a glass of ice chips from the contraption on the fridge door.

"That was so stupid!" Brendon is saying.

"It was an accident," I correct.

"Stupid anyway. Look at the cookies."

"Don't say that, Brendon," Trimble turns to look back at him. "And don't eat those cookies off the floor. Get a broom."

"Trimble's right. Go get a broom," I say and put a towel of ice chips into Sean's red fist. "Poor babe. Come on, we'll go sit in the den."

Trimble and I walk him down the stairs to the den and onto the couch. We kiss him and pat his head while he tries to catch his breath and stop crying, shooting dour looks at his brother.

A part of Sean wants to squirm away and punch him out. I feel him make the effort. "Don't pay attention to Brendon," I say. "He only wants to make you mad." Trimble looks at me, and her eyes are wide and serious and swim with the familiar message: is this normal? "Don't you remember this?" I ask her. She does her Who, me? eyebrow hike, mouth drawn down: no never. Then Sean puts his head in her lap and she turns wistful. Dark Trimble is a moody girl, stirred up easily as water.

She tells me Peter has cried when the shots haven't worked, and sometimes she thinks Peter must regret being saddled with her, a useless, *barren* woman. When I hear about their suffering, I feel helpless, probably in the way Mother said she felt when I told her I was getting a divorce. What can you do?

She looks into the present the boys share and asks, "Do you think they'll be close when they grow up?"

"Oh, yes," I say, believing it, despite their fighting, because I've seen them, conspiring beneath the dining table and because I've found them in the same bed together, talking or asleep, the larger, sidelong and running, one leg tangled in a sheet, the other on his back, tidy package. They are as different asleep as they are awake: the one, even in dreams, in a pant, dodging the many things that chase him; the other, surer, quiet, the fretful bottom of nightmare as terrible as any but far away as sea ground. They are close, these boys, I'm sure of it, and dream what we dreamed, Trimble and I, that our parents would reunite, that we would all be together forever.

Trimble tells me that Peter's older brothers were mean to him, too. "He was so much younger," she says. "Once they took him on a long ride in a wagon. They told him he was adopted and they were taking him to his real parents. He got so scared, he ran half way home before he got lost and had to wait for them to find him." She twists her hair around a finger.

"Maybe that's one of the reasons we're so close," she says and goes on to tell me how on nights before Peter travels, they dance in the den to a Springsteen song. She kisses Sean's head, then gets up to play the song for me. She says, "Listen to the lyrics, now." Brendon comes to sit next to me, and we all three, Brendon, Sean, and I concentrate on the song, but all I see are small towns and battered cars and rummy places where people still smoke cigarettes. I see Peter, too, and Trimble, bumping along together in a rusty wagon. Springsteen's voice opens wide, and my sister, whose face has softened, nudges me.

I say, "If I ever fall in love again, I hope it's as far gone as you two are."

She says, "Oh," and her lower lashes mat with tears.

When we were girls, I used to resent Trimble for crying so often and so easily, almost to occasion it seemed to me then, and I would tease her or frizzle the moment with some cruelty. "It's stupid to cry about Dad; he doesn't love us like his real daughters." Now, when I'm sincere, she turns away, girlish and embarrassed.

I ask Brendon, "Want to dance?" and he gives me a not-on-your-life look, and Sean, sensing he's next, hides behind him, and together they begin to gag on the idea. At least they're friends again. So I walk over to where Trimble is standing, watching the record, and take hold of her hand to dance. Her hand is so warm and familiar, it feels like where we left off. We slow dance, and she flirts with me, sashays around and under my arms. The boys are really whooping it up now. They're pummeling each other with pillows. They're thinking they've never see this before. They're wondering who are these women.

SHARON THESEN

Elegy, The Fertility Specialist _____

He gave it to me straight
and I had to thank him
for the information, the percentages
that dwindled in his pencil writing
hand. I watched them drop
from 70, to 40, to 20
as all the variables were added in
and even after 20 he made a question mark. I felt
doors closing in swift silent succession
as I passed each checkpoint on the way
to the cold awful ruler, expert astronomer,
charterer of heavenly colonies,
answerer of questions, and this question
Could we have a child? and this answer, No
I don't think so. Oh
of course he could go in there
and have a look if I really wanted,
steer his ship around the fraying edges
of my terrain, peering with his spyglass,
cross-hatching impediments on his diagram
of the uterine pear & its two branching filaments:
he wouldn't recommend it, he would say,
squeezing his spyglass shut and putting it back
in its maroon velvet box. We make the usual
small gestures of disappointment
as if we'd run out of luck in a ticket line
and I say goodbye
and walk past the receptionist
busy at her files and it is
as if something with wings was crushing itself
to my heart, to comfort
or to be comforted I didn't know which
or even what it was, some angel, and
entered the elevator with the gabbing nurses
going down to lunch and a little girl
in a sun dress, her delicate
golden shoulders stencilled from the lines
of her bathing suit: a perfect white X.

GLORIA FRYM

Strange Fruit _____

For a long time now every pregnant woman is my enemy.
It's nothing personal, a certain curve magnetizes my eye.
It seems like hatred but it is really sorrow.
He tries to protect me but who protects him.
Fruitless, I contradict what nature intended.
I am a flat thin angle, a dry bud
slapped from the branch. Each birthday
is not enough to have been born. I want to bear. To bear!
But the birds of loss made a nest here.

*

I saw all this happen to her, I witnessed all this, I wasn't her, I was another, her appointed archivist, her medical record, her loyal companion, the angel on her shoulder, a part of we, a child she bore, lost, would have again, but not before accounts were settled. *Christ was no more a man than I am a woman.* An invisible burden, a silk prison, a blood come down, a nothing to show, a desire that weighed so much it held her fast to the earth, face in the mud, muzzled.

*

He's a corporation. He sells hope and dangles it before the desperate. He smiles at discomfort, he implores you to hold still, as your tilted uterus could be the demon. "It has to hurt," and so it does hurt, as he forks his fingers up your openings. He's the one who never looks you in the eye, he's the one you see weekly for six months and he doesn't recognize you walking down the street. He's the one who shrieks, Good Mucous! speaking to sperm he finds in the clear, viscous pool that covers the deeps of you. Each time you catch his pale blue Aryan eye your womb begins to burn as though he were branding you. Now it is already spring. He has felt your breasts and they are ornamental, like those plum trees with the pinkest blossoms, candy-tufted and fragrant but no fruit. Now it is summer again, and you bear no plum.

*

I go to a doctor. He is an old man. He takes me into what looks like a girls' gym with showers and dressing booths. Somehow he gets me on the floor to administer "treatment." I am very embarassed. When it's over and I try to find my clothes, I ask the doctor how many women he's gotten pregnant with this therapy. He tells me a story about a 55 year old woman who wanted a baby. Then I ask him how many others and he doesn't answer. How funny to have kids come out looking like him, thinking they'll look like him as an old man when they are born.

*

To be pregnant, in Spanish: embarazada. But monuments to Maternidad everywhere. Stone voluptuaries with large laps full of infant, white breasts bulging from bodices of marble dress. Go deep into the tropics to heat the cold stove, Isla Mujeres where Felix was conceived, his mother wanted him so. In the airport, every Mexican woman surrounded by several children, and one in the oven, a group of embarazadas travelling like a junta, bellies leading the way. The years have done to Isla what they've done to my womb: something's moved in and taken over. Palm tree blight, great brown fronds line the soapy shore, gone birds, against lonely aquamarine.

*

I begin to grow younger and younger. Wanting the child, I become the child, until I am the child, crying easily and without language. Wanting mother. Then the morning newspaper robbing us both of any innocence we might have accumulated during the night. Silence took me like a disease, silence mistook me for a quiet one who knows her place. Dismembered confidence, unfit for reception, no conception. As though everything I am had another, better life apart from me. Buckets of water balanced on my shoulders. Where to pour what I worked to fill. Heavier than solid, but contained as an object. Childless mother, a sac within filled with potential yous. They're all a brew, but the woman's shoe is different than the shoe without a woman.

*

She says just relax and take these Women's Precious Pills and try a little Tai Chi and love yourself more and a few acupuncture treatments and forgive yourself and then some homeopathic doses no coffee what a pity don't let them take anything out of you Western Medicine just visualize Rolfe your Body Have a Happy Life Be Kind Be Well You're a Lovely Mess.

*

Slippery secret of the wet nest where origin generates. A fern pattern, a plan fills the lens. One sticky drop of elastic sea, translucent for three days. He observes his germ, and he is confirmed by the single swimming thing, amphibious aggressor off to find my queen, on its way to the mouth of the canal where she hatches another slow plot. I am the element in which it moves, aquatic, uncertain of my queen's decision. Sweet lady of the dark forest, the path is clear, grant our wish.

*

Monthly report from the province of the interior. Blood is the language, words are the cells, phrases clot. Troops of sperm living and dying to meet their half. Isn't the love big enough? Aren't we the picture perfect? Didn't we do it right, dog style this time, then turn me over and legs up so as not to spill a drop? Won't it take, why didn't it take, are we allergic? Is my baggage too heavy, am I sick with disease? Are there reasons for this? As though statistics chose their hostage. No one we love can't do this. My work now impossible because I cannot give him what I am made to give him. Am I made to give?

But I want to give. I am not my body, after all. I am more than my body, the one who lives behind the beehive, inside, curled, childless, without childhood to relive through a another. The one and the two and the other. That other I can't seem to make. I cannot make the One who could be separate.

Now that I am separating from Her.

*

I am with a doctor who has just taken some X-rays of my spine. The doctor turns to me and says, I have some very interesting information for you—you were born two girls.

*

Trying becomes a career. But there is no dress for success, only jets of the possible soaring then crashing then reassembling, like cartoon figures smashing against a wall and walking through the other side. This goes on for years, morning thermometer like a strange glass cigarette, a life is charted by the body's temperature, by the rise and fall of fever. This sickness replaces all other desire. Timed loved tires the love. Pee into cup, add white powder, wait twenty minutes, add blue powder, wait for color change, measure color against chart color, are we ready? We want to look inside, we want to see the exact release of egg into the expanding universe! Plant a little camera there and wait. Instead, day 13, ultrasound, doctor sticks dick shaped microphone up twat, microphone wears rubber, rubber wears jelly, his hand on my belly, sound making a frizzy picture on a screen. See that follicle, he screams, it's a beauty! Go home and do it tonight.

*

—Mommy, how did I get to be a baby in your stomach?
—Daddy put a seed there and you grew in me.
—But Mommy, how did he get the seed in your stomach?
(Mother clears throat with resignation.)
—Well, he put his penis in my vagina, and a seed came out of his penis.
—Mommy, I'm serious, don't joke with me.

*

She's the Specialist, Hormones are Her, she's the hot number you pick like a lotto ticket and wait six months to get the scoop. She's the one you'll let cut into you, small white hands make a better surgeon. And she's the excellent one. Stakes her claim like Cortez with a small band of pale soldiers we all think are gods. But she's the one who wears boxy nun shoes, and speaks in Spartan tones. She's an Assistant Professor, on her way to Full Professor. She's the one who asks for money up front, she's the one who sees you like a 15 minute whore, then washes her hands of you.

*

Newborn left under sink in airplane bathroom, newborn left on front steps of Church of the Epiphany wearing LA Raider's jacket and socks on his hands and feet, newborn found under liquid amber in Golden Gate Park late November, covered by red leaves, Moses in the bullrushes, appears to be healthy, appears to be abandoned, appears to be motherless, fatherless, homeless, without a country, newly minted, newly arrived, newly exiled, unclaimed, unwanted, unplanned, unharmed, alive. Not mine.

*

Because Psyche looked at Love square in the face, Love said, you can't have a Divine Child.

*

He's the one who reviews medical records like pulp novels. He's the one who never touches you. He's the one with preprinted scripts for the miracle drug. He's the one who says a higher dose makes you more yourself. He's the one who never leaves his desk, pipe smoke against a book-lined backdrop, for $300 an hour your own vanity press. Still behind the desk, he rises like a president to shake your hand. He's the one who always seems to be out of town during anyone's ovulation. So up the dose! Little side effects, little suicidal defects are normal. Can't tolerate? Then Anesthetize! Repair the tube, spare the rod. Cut out the cells, clean up the whole garage. Patch the tire, put in some 50 weight oil man, and sell her quick.

*

All desire translated into what we could not have. Baby shoes, small animals, infant sorrow. All we could not have. The whole world seemed to have what we could not have, had too much of what we could not have, had too many of what we could not have, even abused what we could not have. We believed in justice, as gamblers believe they'll always win against the odds. Our minds fell out of our bodies and we craved our reward. We could remember when we did not desire this, when every month held the reverse terror. This desire, which was visceral, did not embody thought, but reaction. A nausea, a vertigo, as in pregnancy.

*

Driving long distances, I think I'm pregnant, but I'm just having an out of the car experience. The road starts to enter the car as the car absorbs the road, and I feel pleasantly off balance, as though I were finally part of my surroundings.

*

I'm lying on the examining table, waiting for the doctor to finish a pregnancy test. He's putting a handful of footlong Q-tips into a solution, one at a time. He does each one individually, methodically. He's warning me to do something about the course I'm on, and he announces that I'm not pregnant. Then he comes over to the table and leans over and attempts to kiss me. I push him away, telling him he shouldn't do that, especially in my situation.

*

Having exhausted all methods of conjure, having put gold rings at the feet of the Chinese goddess of mercy, having lit three blue candles each day for the right number of days, having faith, having believed, having felt the requisite swell, loosened the cinch, kept the company of correspondent beings, wished on hailstones, burned myrrh, consumed heat, swallowed bitter herbs—now put a piece of paper in the typewriter and command the typist to type, as you might switch on the player piano and begin the music without the musician.

*

Just before we give up, not being able to as real as being able to. Wake up at two hour intervals, feeding something that does not yet exist, change habits as though the sun had permanently shifted in me, a kind of long winter sets in and I stay close to home. Dreams of the child who will seem to pick us, just us, out of the universe.

*

I have a baby, but didn't know I was pregnant. When I had a pregnancy test it came out negative. I didn't even gain weight. The baby is wonderful, Summer is here and we put the baby on a bed, tuck her in and make some food for her. It occurs to me that I might have some milk. I take out my left breast and squeeze the nipple but nothing comes, then I take out the right breast and put it in the baby's mouth. She sucks and I'm very happy. She is very hungry and eats almost every hour and cries just a tiny bit.

*

We are told to ask ourselves Why. As though reason would make it happen, or stall the inevitable. In the deepest place, there is no reason. Desire to do, without reason, as in the beginning, as a child, with play.

Now the years have manufactured reason, and the factory never closes. The desire to name and name that which one bears and claim it from a certain chaos, this most natural desire. That's Why. Stronger than first love, than sex, than pleasure, than hunger, stronger than sacrifice —this monthly blood, still ripping out the heart with a dull knife.

*

We bought a ticket to Paris but the plane takes us to Madrid.
We bought a ticket to London but the plane takes us to Stockholm.
We bought a ticket around the world but instead we fall into a
deep sleep and dream our entire lives backwards, as though
retracing our desires, as though desire were a place.
We go to Hawaii and notice everyone speaks Spanish there. We're
in luck! We speak Spanish better than French.
We rent a tiny house. The furniture seems built for very small
people, but when we sit down, it fits us perfectly.
We apologize for all this strange fruit.
We collapse into the sofa, heaving great thunderous sobs
as though at last the gods had touched us.

*

This child will create herself. By silent instructions, and the other secret she finds by being born. That I could not hold this one inside, my grief. But that I could take one to be mine to protect, my pleasure. Child who could not be mothered by another, come to me, I who did not have a mother, others took me for their own, also.

The largest grief will paint itself into the longest beauty. Desire at last modified, as in expansion. That abstraction, into a particular body. A child! Who is our own rebirth. Darling, I'm waiting for you to find me.

ANAÏS NIN

Birth _____

"The child," said the doctor, "is dead."

I lay stretched on a table. I had no place on which to rest my legs. I had to keep them raised. Two nurses leaned over me. In front of me stood the doctor with the face of a woman and eyes protruding with anger and fear. For two hours I had been making violent efforts. The child inside of me was six months old and yet it was too big for me. I was exhausted, the veins in me were swelling with the strain. I had pushed with my entire being. I had pushed as if I wanted this child out of my body and hurled into another world.

"Push, push with all your strength!"

Was I pushing with all my strength? All my strength?

No. A part of me did not want to push out the child. The doctor knew it. That is why he was angry, mysteriously angry. He knew. A part of me lay passive, did not want to push out anyone, not even this dead fragment of myself, out in the cold, outside of me. All in me which chose to keep, to lull, to embrace, to love, all in me which carried, preserved, and protected, all in me which imprisoned the whole world in its passionate tenderness, this part of me would not thrust out the child, even though it had died in me. Even though it threatened my life, I could not break, tear out, separate, surrender, open and dilate and yield up a fragment of a life like a fragment of the past, this part of me rebelled against pushing out the child, or anyone, out in the cold, to be picked up by strange hands, to be buried in strange places, to be lost, lost, lost. . . . He knew, the doctor. A few hours before he adored me, served me. Now he was angry. And I was angry with a black anger at this part of me which refused to push, to separate, to lose.

"Push! Push! Push with all your strength!"

I pushed with anger, with despair, with frenzy, with the feeling that I would die pushing, as one exhales the last breath, that I would push out everything inside of me, and my soul with all the blood around it, and the sinews with my heart inside of them, choked, and that my body itself would open and smoke would rise, and I would feel the ultimate incision of death.

The nurses leaned over me and they talked to each other while I rested. Then I pushed until I heard my bones cracking, until my veins swelled. I closed my eyes so hard I saw lightning and waves of red and purple. There was a stir in my ears, a beating as if the tympanum would burst. I closed my lips so tightly the blood was trickling. My legs felt enormously heavy, like marble columns, like immense marble columns crushing my body. I was pleading for someone to hold them. The nurse laid her knee on my stomach and shouted: "Push! Push! Push!" Her perspiration fell on me.

The doctor paced up and down angrily, impatiently. "We will be here all night. Three hours now. . . ."

The head was showing, but I had fainted. Everything was blue, then black. The instruments were gleaming before my eyes. Knives sharpened in my ears. Ice and silence. Then I heard voices, first talking too fast for me to understand. A curtain was parted, the voices still tripped over each other, falling fast like a waterfall, with sparks, and cutting into my ears. The table was rolling gently, rolling. The women were lying in the air. Heads. Heads hung where the enormous white bulbs of the lamps were hung. The doctor was still walking, the lamps moved, the heads came near, very near, and the words came more slowly.

They were laughing. One nurse was saying: "When I had my first child I was all ripped to pieces. I had to be sewn up again, and then I had another, and had to be sewn up, and then I had another. . . ."

The other nurse said: "Mine passed like an envelope through a letter box. But afterwards the bag would not come out. The bag would not come out. Out. Out. . . ." Why did they keep repeating themselves. And the lamps turning. And the steps of the doctor very fast, very fast.

"She can't labor any more, at six months nature does not help. She should have another injection."

I felt the needle thrust. The lamps were still. The ice and the blue that was all around came into my veins. My heart beat wildly. The nurses talked: "Now that baby of Mrs. L. last week, who would have thought she was too small, a big woman like that, a big woman like that, a big woman like that. . . ." The words kept turning, as on a disk. They talked, they talked, they talked. . . ."

Please hold my legs! Please hold my legs! Please hold my legs! PLEASE HOLD MY LEGS! I am ready again. By throwing my head back I can see the clock. I have been struggling four hours. It would be better to die. Why am I alive and struggling so desperately? I could not remember why I should want to live. I could not remember anything. Everything was blood and pain. I have to push. I have to push. That is a black fixed point in eternity. At the end of a long dark tunnel. I have to push. A voice saying: "Push! Push! Push!" A knee on my stomach and the marble of my legs crushing me and the head so large and I have to push.

Am I pushing or dying? The light up there, the immense round blazing white light is drinking me. It drinks me slowly, inspires me into space. If I do not close my eyes it will drink all of me. I seep upward, in long icy threads, too light, and yet inside there is a fire too, the nerves are twisted, there is no rest from this long tunnel dragging me, or am I pushing myself out of the tunnel, or is the child being pushed out of me, or is the light drinking me. Am I dying? The ice in the veins, the cracking of the bones, this pushing in darkness, with a small shaft of light in the eyes like the edge of a knife, the feeling of a knife cutting the flesh, the flesh somewhere is tearing as if it were burned through by a flame, somewhere my flesh is tearing and the blood is spilling out. I am pushing in the darkness, in utter darkness. I am pushing until my eyes open and I see the doctor holding a long instrument which he swiftly thrusts into me and the pain makes me cry out. A long animal howl. That will make her push, he says to the nurse. But it does not. It paralyzes me with pain. He wants to do it again. I sit up with fury and I shout at him: "Don't you dare do that again, don't you dare!"

The heat of my anger warms me, all the ice and pain are melted in the fury. I have an instinct that what he has done is unnecessary, that he has done it because he is in a rage, because the hands on the clock keep turning, the dawn is coming and the child does not come out, and I am losing strength and the injection does not produce the spasm.

I look at the doctor pacing up and down, or bending to look at the head which is barely showing. He looks baffled, as before a savage mystery, baffled by this struggle. He wants to interfere with his instruments, while I struggle with nature, with myself, with my child and with the meaning I put into it all, with my desire to give and to hold, to keep and to lose, to live and to die. No instrument can help me. His eyes are furious. He would like to take a knife. He has to watch and wait.

I want to remember all the time why I should want to live. I am all pain and no memory. The lamp has ceased drinking me. I am too weary to move even towards the light, or to turn my head and look at the clock. Inside of my body there are fires, there are bruises, the flesh is in pain. The child is not a child, it is a demon strangling me. The demon lies inert at the door of the womb, blocking life, and I cannot rid myself of it.

The nurses begin to talk again. I say: let me alone. I put my two hands on my stomach and very softly, with the tips of my fingers I drum drum drum drum drum drum on my stomach in circles. Around, around, softly, with eyes open in great serenity. The doctor comes near with amazement on his face. The nurses are silent. Drum drum drum drum drum drum in soft circles, soft quiet circles. Like a savage. The mystery. Eyes open, nerves begin to shiver, ... a mysterious agitation. I hear the ticking of the clock ... inexorably, separately. The little nerves awake, stir. But my hands are so weary, so weary, they will fall off. The womb is stirring and dilating. Drum drum drum drum drum. I am ready! The nurse presses her knee on my stomach. There is blood in my eyes. A tunnel. I push into this tunnel, I bite my lips and push. There is a fire and flesh ripping and no air. Out of the tunnel! All my blood is spilling out. Push! Push! Push! It is coming! It is coming! It is coming! I feel the slipperiness, the sudden deliverance, the weight is gone. Darkness. I hear voices. I open my eyes. I hear them saying: "It was a little girl. Better not show it to her." All my strength returns. I sit up. The doctor shouts: "Don't sit up!"

"Show me the child!"

"Don't show it," says the nurse, "it will be bad for her." The nurses try to make me lie down. My heart is beating so loud I can hardly hear myself repeating: "Show it to me." The doctor holds it up. It looks dark and small, like a diminutive man. But it is a little girl. It has long eyelashes on its closed eyes, it is perfectly made, and all glistening with the waters of the womb.

oo oo oo

RACHEL BLAU DUPLESSIS

Undertow _____

That I am rigid   dead in a sheet
awake
the night melting   my body melting
my head   rock   stark
and hoarding iron

That you have touched my nipple and
I am ripped away with grief

nothing can enter   an empty gulf

Sleek earth, rust brown, a shining
I am driving past this
silent
thru the fog of asking
again and again
what I am severed from.

The undertow
that happens
frozen time   happens
within
rigid
force it pulls me down dead set.
Against.
Battlefield.
My staring   helmeted face
stock still
and desolation

snapped off trees
infertile mud
the uprooted.
My place.
I am the grief.

The undertow
sucks me down
my breath rock hard
under the quick water.

Sleep   pleasure   the open voice   these   it cannot bear
these
powerful   a tide   running out
these   these
that happen
tonight
that cannot happen,
locked
close
the earth
rich
fissure.

Pebble dirt
bare road
cannot move
in bed   that place   cannot
in my breasts   it is finished

Comes
the undertow

not   not   not
myself
is it myself?

oo oo oo

MARIANNE GINGHER

Camouflage _____

She was only sixteen, and hers was a difficult labor with complications. Earlier that afternoon, when the contractions had started, Mary sat on the divan, calmly timing them by the mantel clock, waiting for her mother to emerge from her bedroom, perhaps take charge. Her mother was drunk. Finally Mary called Alexia, her older sister, and it was Alexia who drove her to the hospital and held her hand off and on all night until the doctor ordered a Caesarean. Alexia kept taking cigarette breaks for which she apologized, but Mary was secretly glad whenever Alexia slipped away. She relished the chance to die—for surely she was dying—without frightening anybody who knew her. Whenever Alexia left the labor room, Mary screamed. She was sick and tired of bravery.

The baby was normal—that's all the doctor told her. A girl with reddish hair. The doctor lay the child casually on Mary's chest as if Mary were a shelf. Instinctively she touched the top of the baby's sticky head and felt life beating furiously: the eager, steamy warmth of it, the warmth dissipating into the cool, stoic air of the delivery room. She longed to cradle the child against herself but felt too shy. She wanted to press it against the cavelike void of who she'd been once. Who was she now? She wanted the child to make some sort of difference, to heal her from her vague, repentant self. What did she have to repent now that it was over? The baby lay upon her, soft and pink like gathered flowers. When she began to cry, a nurse scooped her up and swaddled her in towels. Mary never saw her again.

She slept a sleep like falling: there was pain when she hit bottom. She awoke, crying from the pain of her incision, but also crying from some darkly unimpeachable center of herself where she knew her suffering was for nothing. A nurse brought her medication and she slept until late morning. She dreamed that Jim Davenport stood over her bed with a paper cone of flowers. In her dream he was as old as her father. He combed his thinning hair backwards, and you could see the furrows left by the comb. He talked of bank loans and car repairs and where you could still get a good shoeshine cheaply. He talked as if she were on his list of things to do.

Yet, when she awoke, she half-expected him to be there. She'd known he wouldn't be, known he never would be again. Still, she kept wishing for him—it was the only thing that made her heart feel alive. If only the doctor had been able to deliver her from foolishness, too.

You got rid of your innocence, but that was nothing, really, in the great foolish scheme of your life.

She couldn't eat breakfast. Looking at the tray nauseated her. She drank a few tentative sips of hot tea. The epidural hadn't worn off, and she wasn't allowed to sit up. A nurse helped her with a sponge bath.

Around eleven o'clock Alexia appeared with their mother. Mrs. Spencer was wearing dark glasses that she didn't take off. Her smile wobbled, but she bent and kissed Mary lightly on the cheek and handed her a heart-shaped package with a glamorous pink bow.

"How are you feeling today, hon?" Alexia asked, brushing her hand across Mary's brow in a motherly, fever-testing way. She'd bought a *People* magazine in the lobby and placed it on top of Mary's bedside table. One of the buttons on her car coat was missing and so she'd fastened the coat together with a diaper pin. She looked tired, ragged. She was nearly thirty, with three young children and a husband who traveled during the week. She patted Mary's hand. "Life will get back to normal now. You'll see."

It was what Mary wished her mother would say. But her mother only walked to the window, parted the shade and looked out, silent. Her mother didn't act like a mother anymore. It was like she'd given up: there had been one disappointment too many. She walked haltingly, like an invalid.

Most days her mother slept until noon. She hardly cooked anymore. For her supper she ate ice cream out of a paper carton and drank a glass of sweet sherry. She never argued. If something disturbed or angered her, she'd retreat to her bedroom and cry. She'd hardly said a word about Mary's pregnancy. She'd neither condemned nor consoled. When Mary had tried to talk with her, she'd stared out the nearest window as if she were dreaming up a plan, as if advice were on the tip of her tongue if she could only order her thoughts. She'd acted aloof, and, considering her circumstances, it had been easy to mistake her aloofness for courage.

But Mary had looked out windows, too, into the bleak, resourceless night of her decision, enduring Alexia's heartless wisdom. "It's a family tradition," Alexia had said. "Husband *then* baby."

The nurse came in and gave Mary two pills: one for discomfort and one to dry up her breast milk. "What a pretty package!" the nurse exclaimed. "Now that should cheer you up."

Mary's mother turned from the window and smiled. But the smile had no energy source. It came from nowhere and went nowhere like a statue's.

"Open it, Mary," Alexia said.

She drew the heart-shaped package into her lap and loosened the ribbon. It was candy: expensive-looking chocolates wrapped in golden foil. The sort of gift that reminded her that her mother didn't know how to go about knowing her, the sort of gift that unleashed unexpected sadness. She'd already opened Pandora's box, hadn't she? Last April in the backseat of Jim Davenport's car. The awful surprise of how easily it had happened. She'd thought of sex as some sort of complicated contraption that she could never fathom: too many nuts and bolts to unloosen, too many opportunities to be clumsy, to wreck the mission, snared zippers, tangled straps. She'd believed that passion required dexterity. But passion had grown its own quick fingers, appendages that bloomed magically in exquisitely empowered places.

Nobody felt like talking, but Alexia tried. She tried to avoid talking about her children, but Alexia wasn't very good at talking about other things. She brought out a piece of quilting from her handbag and talked about that. In a little while, she excused herself to the lobby, where she could smoke.

"Well," Mary's mother said, sitting down in a chair, folding her hands together. "Why do you suppose Alexia smokes? *I* never smoked."

There seemed nothing to talk about because everything was known. Mary tried to guess the weather, thinking that her mother's dark glasses were a clue. "Is it sunny out?" she asked, feeling stupid and inadequate.

Her mother started to cry. "How can you forget all this?" she said. "You'll have that awful scar."

After Alexia and her mother left, two girlfriends, Bev and Lisa, dropped by. They were the only friends she'd kept up with since she dropped out of school that fall. They brought flowers and ate the chocolate candy and turned on the television to watch a tennis match. They'd gone to the Homecoming Dance on Saturday night, the night Mary was having the baby. They said the dance was "pathetic." Mr. Houston, the machine shop teacher, and Miss Keck, the art teacher, had gone out to dinner before the dance and gotten wasted. Then, they'd fallen all over each other, dancing at the gym. They'd done the Dirty Dog and the assistant principal had made them leave. They'd probably get fired.

A lot of the students had come to the dance drunk or stoned. Some sophomore boys got arrested in the bathroom for fighting, ripping toilet seats off their hinges and using them for weapons. Everybody said that David Cannon and Jim Davenport were so stoned that they traversed the entire school parking lot by jumping from car hood to car hood. "Oh, *sorry,*" Bev said, casting Mary a guilty look. "I guess it's pretty tacky of us to mention Jim Davenport."

"He didn't bring a date," Lisa said in a conciliatory way. "And he looked totally miserable." She popped a piece of chocolate candy in her mouth and leaned toward the television. "What a bod," she said to the tennis player.

"Who got crowned Homecoming Queen?" Mary asked.

They made similar faces of disgust. "Candace Yardley," they said in mincing, jeerful voices. "The dream whore."

Whore. The word seemed to darken the room like the curse of an uninvited witch. But Mary saw by their bland, unremorseful expressions that Bev and Lisa hadn't heard what they'd said. How pure and changeless they were. Mary laughed, but not for the reason they thought. She felt *relieved* that all of it was lost to her. It had been lost to her while she was pregnant, but in a different way: the kind of losing in which what's gone is gone but you still yearn for it. Now, hearing about the Homecoming Dance, she felt absolved. Her baby seemed a living, breathing talisman against all trivia. Even Jim Davenport. Especially Jim Davenport.

"Jim Davenport," she said stonily, and her friends looked at her. "Jim Davenport. Krispy Kreme. Mello-Yello. Disneyland. King Kong."

Her father had been out of town on business, and since his divorce from her mother his contact was infrequent at best. He said he wouldn't have even known about the delivery if he hadn't bumped into Mary's mother in the grocery store. "So she told me," he said, shaking his head. "Right there in the grocery store while she examined apples for bruises. 'Oh, by the way, Fred,' she says, 'it's over.' " He sighed ruefully. " 'A head of lettuce, a dozen eggs, a baby.' "

Mary squirmed beneath her sheet.

"She didn't really say it like that," he said.

"Please, Daddy," Mary said, but she was glad to have him there and didn't give her request the force of a protest. It was a cajoling voice she used, so wry it made him smile.

He kissed her on the forehead.

He was only forty-eight, but he had a sober, grandfatherly air, sitting on the edge of her bed, his shoulders stooped, his hair silver and wispily receding from his forehead. The gold-rimmed glasses he wore gave him a fragile look. When he leaned forward to kiss her, she smelled the professionally starched aroma of his shirt. He always carried a handkerchief in his pocket. When she missed him most, she missed the way he smelled, smells that evoked sensations of ritual and order: shoe polish and aftershave and cinnamon-flavored toothpicks.

He held her hands for a moment, rubbing them, and then in an odd, congratulatory voice he said, "At least you didn't marry your mistake."

That night she thought a lot about her mistake. She supposed she should hate the baby now, hate how it had changed her life. But she didn't hate it, had never hated it. The truth was that having the baby had made her feel bolder and expansive. She was not just herself anymore. From now on she was herself *and* a baby, filling up two places in the world, not one. They would be absent from each other but never alone. Invisible threads of love would always connect them.

The counselor from the Crisis Pregnancy Center had come by the hospital to talk with her, encourage her to express her anger and sorrow forthrightly. When Mary could only talk about the invisible threads of love, the counselor looked concerned. When had she decided to give the baby up? Whose decision had it finally been? Alexia's? Her father's? Mr. and Mrs. Davenport's? Her own? All she remembered was that the decision had been made long before she ever held the baby. There was every reason in the world to give the baby up except one: its quickening luster as it lay upon her at delivery, its power to make her feel necessary.

Nights in the hospital when she couldn't sleep, Mary imagined that her body was telling her that somewhere her baby was wakeful, too. She envisioned its adoptive mother slipping on a bathrobe to warm milk for a late-night feeding. The mother held the baby in a room silvered with moonlight and the milk had a sweet, flowerlike scent. The woman who held the baby was learning to love it. She'd been wanting a child for many years and Mary had granted her a miracle.

In this way, thinking about what the pregnancy counselor had said, Mary calmed herself and didn't feel expendable. Sometimes she even pitied the adoptive mother whom she imagined feared the baby in the dead of night, feared its insatiable needs and eventual understanding, perhaps wondering if she could ever love it enough. For it seemed to Mary that the baby would almost expect to be loved more by a woman who was not its natural mother and yet had so fiercely chosen to rear it. That a child would be infinitely comforted by the knowledge that it was no accident in the life of such a person.

Then, on the last day of her hospital stay, when no visitors came to distract her, Mary began to believe that she'd made a terrible mistake, giving the baby away. That it was the baby she needed more than anything else to help her distinguish what truly mattered from what did not.

She was released from the hospital on Thanksgiving Day. Bruce, Alexia's husband, came to get her and drove her straight to their house where Alexia was making Thanksgiving dinner. Mary's mother was already there, sitting in the den, watching a Snoopy cartoon special with the children. She waved at Mary from the sofa and smiled her distant smile.

Alexia threw her arms around Mary and made a big deal of her arrival. "Look how skinny you already are!" Alexia cried. "It's always taken me six months to get my figure back." She was drinking a glass of wine and she poured one for Mary. "Cheers!" she said.

They'd never been particularly close, Alexia and Mary. They were thirteen years apart. But Mary sensed a new bond now, the sort of bond in which Alexia acknowledged Mary's adulthood in the generous-spirited way of friends rather than with the investigatory rivalry of sisters. They were actually drinking wine together; it felt peculiar and cozy.

Mary sat on a kitchen stool and chopped up celery for the salad. Bruce carved the turkey so attentively that it looked as if he were repairing something. Each slice was paper-thin, and Alexia was so pleased that she threw her arms around his waist. "Hey, you'll mess me up," he said.

"I'd love to mess you up," Alexia said with a low, throaty laugh, and they exchanged an intimate look.

Bruce laughed at her. "Better watch the wine," he cautioned.

Alexia reached for the bottle defiantly and sloshed out another rosy glassful. She held it up and stared at it intently until Bruce noticed. "What are you doing *now*?"

"I'm *watching* the wine," she said.

Bruce put down the carving knife, grabbed her wrist and pulled her against him. They kissed a long time until finally Mary left the kitchen. She felt light-headed, squirmy with embarrassment. It was too warm in the kitchen, too suddenly sentimental. It felt like Bruce and Alexia were cooking valentines for dinner. They seemed on display to her, their behavior, like Alexia's sterling flatware, reserved for special occasions only.

Most of the time Bruce was gone, traveling. And so often she'd heard Alexia say that he had a short fuse, sounded off at her and the kids for the least infraction. Nothing very passionate or romantic ever came to mind when she thought of Alexia's marriage. They had money enough, but Alexia didn't seem to care. She spent the money on furniture and forgot about the way she looked. She dressed like a slob and her hair was a mess. She ran around in a shabby, unstylish coat fastened with a diaper pin, taking care of kids with chicken pox, coping alone. With Bruce away, Alexia slept alone five nights a week. What had she been after in the first place and where had it gotten to?

Mary slipped on her coat and walked out into the backyard to the swing set. She slumped down on the sliding board and her hips just fit within the narrow borders. She began to think about her baby. But her sense of the baby was different now than it had been at the hospital. What would she have named it? "Christabel," she said aloud, as if to make the baby more real. Already she could feel the whole experience slipping beyond her, the invisible threads of love thinning. She could almost imagine that it had never happened, and it seemed that the rest of them were eager for her to forget. Chopping celery in the kitchen, talking about getting her figure back, hearing the comforting hum of the Snoopy show in the background, giving birth had begun to seem like just another kind of domestic event. First you are in one place, then another, misfortune simply part of the landscape of travel. That simple. Having a baby had been like stopping off for a minute in a ghost town. You certainly couldn't get off the bus and stay. There was nothing for you there, so you just rode on and you didn't ask where.

"Christabel," she said again. Why had she thought of such a name? It came from something she'd read at school. Some poem. It sounded antique and breakable. Sweep up the pieces and throw them away.

Alexia opened the back door. "You feeling okay, Mary?" She could tell by the casualness of Alexia's tone that they expected her to act weird. "Eke's coming out to join you," Alexia called cheerfully.

That's right, Mary thought, pretend to the crazy person that you think she's normal as pie.

Eke hopped down the back stoop wearing the roller skates she practically slept in and her Walkman. She was ten years old, Alexia's only daughter. Her real name was Ethyl, the same as Bruce's mother. Eke liked to say that when she first heard her name, after she'd quit gagging, she'd screamed "Eeek!" She skated expertly across the wintry grass and flopped, belly first, into a swing beside Mary.

"Want some gum?" she asked, digging into a pocket of her skintight jeans. She had long, brittle-looking, coltish legs. She gouged out a piece of Bazooka.

"Thanks." Mary opened the gum and read the fortune aloud: " 'Love conquers all.' "

Eke sneered. "I hate fortunes like that. It's like the pamphlets they give you at Sunday school. It's like the damn Care Bears."

"*Please*," Mary said. "My stitches. It still hurts when I laugh."

"Mom sent me out to tell you dinner's almost ready," Eke said. "You want to listen to the Pre-Minstrels first?" She took off her headphones and offered them to Mary. "This group is monumentally sick," she said fondly.

Mary put the headphones on and listened for a while.

"Bet you think they're called the Pre-Minstrels because of PMS, right?" Eke said, grinning. "Wrong. They're called the Pre-Minstrels because none of them have started their periods yet. These chicks are all eleven years old. And foxy."

"They sound a little like Madonna," Mary said, thinking she was being complimentary, but Eke made a face and looked insulted.

When Mary took the headphones off, Eke said more softly, "I'm sorry you couldn't keep the baby. Mom said it was a girl." Eke shook her head and gestured toward the house where her younger brothers were still watching cartoons. "Boys are such a pain," she said. "Damn," she said, "a girl sure would have been nice."

They ate Thanksgiving dinner on Alexia's new dining room table with Queen Anne legs. Alexia acted nervous. She made the two boys eat with their fingers rather than utensils they might use to bang on the new table. One spilled his milk, and after she'd mopped up the spot with a damp cloth, she brought out furniture polish, too. The bitter smell of the polish sickened Mary and she excused herself.

"Go lie down in Eke's room," Alexia said kindly. "I know you must feel worn out, hon."

Eke's room was painted black. Neon-colored posters of rock stars papered the ceiling. A mishmash of bumper stickers plastered the wall above her bed: ARMS ARE FOR HUGGING. IF YOU CAN READ THIS GET OFF MY ASS. LIFE SUCKS AND THEN YOU DIE. On the bed lay a worn-out Raggedy Ann doll, her hair restyled in a Mohawk, her skirt trimmed to mini length. She had diaper pins for earrings.

Mary stretched across the bed, closing her eyes, but she couldn't fall asleep. Downstairs voices praised the meal. She could hear the twinkling babble of china and silverware, ice rattling in glasses, sounds so reassuring and homey that she felt gathered-in. For the first time in a long while her heart felt quiet; she was back in Little Girl Land. She would go to the private Catholic school across town like her father wanted. He would pay the tuition, and she would make new friends. Her past wouldn't follow her. She'd forget the invisible threads of love. She'd stop wearing makeup, let all the blond grow out of her hair. Cut her hair short. Cut her fingernails and resume piano lessons. Make good grades. She'd be a better friend to Eke, help Alexia more with the kids. She'd invite her mother to go to the movies. They'd take old-fashioned dancing lessons together at Fred Astaire. They'd dance *together*, no men.

It exhausted her to think about all the possibilities, the choices. Pick a card, any card: the magic trick of life. She felt dizzy the way shopping for pantyhose always made her feel dizzy. There seemed an overwhelming amount to decide: not just color and size but seamed or seamless, textured or non-textured, control top, sandal-foot, reinforced toe, cotton crotch. Why should variety blow your circuits? Why should choice feel like punishment? Maybe she was crazy. Maybe you couldn't go through what she'd been through without going crazy. Her hands felt for the spot on her chest where the baby's weight had rested. She couldn't remember, not the color or the size. She pressed her chest until it hurt.

The door cracked open suddenly and Eke poked her head into the room.

"I'm not asleep, it's okay," Mary said.

"I caught a fly for the Lord," Eke said, skating over to the window ledge.

Mary thought she'd heard wrong and sat up.

"I-doo-widdy-caught-a-fly-she-bop-she-bop. I-doo-widdy-caught-a-fly-for-the-Lord," Eke sang.

"Did I die?" Mary said. "Is this heaven or hell?"

Eke laughed. "He's my lizard," she said. "Actually my *anole*, if you want to get technical." She opened a small plastic cage and released the fly she'd caught. "Lord *Alien*," she said softly, unabashedly tender the way children are around animals they love. Her broad goofy smile, with its missing teeth, gentled her, made her spiked, carrot-colored hair and earrings seem an illusion, a special effect.

She set the plastic box on the bed and they watched Lord Alien stalk and devour the fly. "He likes you, Mary," Eke said knowingly, pressing her lips on the cage as if to kiss the lizard. "He's putting on his happy suit."

Obligingly the lizard turned from a mottled brown color to the luminous green of a blade of grass. Eke laughed and said, "He's a dude. Work out with him, Mary." She put the cage in Mary's lap.

"What do I do?"

"Just be his friend. Sing him a song. He likes reptile music."

Mary giggled. "Such as?"

"Try 'Glow Little Glow Worm'—Grandmother Spencer sings that to him. Or 'Puff the Magic Dragon.' Now *that* one inspires him."

Mary tried to imagine her mother singing to the anole and wondered if she'd been drunk. She sang one verse of "Puff the Magic Dragon" but felt silly.

"Look at him eyeballing you," Eke said. "He acts like he's in complete control."

"He's got no choice," Mary said, leaning closer to study him. She felt a swooning sensation. His beauty seemed remote and powerful. He knew absolutely who he was. She was astonished by his feet, so fragile and digital, the long toes—if that was what they were really called—almost transparent, splayed, his little haunches resting on a leaf, positioned the way puppies cooled themselves on the floor in hot weather. His color was that livid green of the objects she had always imagined were most alive: big gracious summer trees, ferns that thickened early in the woods. His scales were as tiny and metallic as dots of dime store glitter. All the while she gazed at him, his own eyes swiveled at odd angles to detect and diminish surprise. "He has *ribs*," Mary said reverently. "I want to hold him."

Eke scooped him quickly from the leaf and drew her hand slowly from the cage. "He's really freaking," she said.

Mary slipped her hands around Eke's and felt the cool, sticky flesh of the anole fluttering against her palms. Carefully Eke withdrew her hand and Mary clasped her palms together, upright, prayerful. The lizard's head poked out between her thumbs. "Hello there," she said. "You're a dude."

"One good squeeze and he'd be lizard soup," Eke said.

"I'll put him back now," Mary said. She felt unaccountably sad. The lizard made her feel bigger than she had a right to be.

Eke fed him a couple of mealworms, in honor of Thanksgiving, then Lord Alien crept under a slab of bark and turned gray. He looked exhausted, or maybe Mary was. She flopped across the bed, and Eke went outside to rollerskate.

Mary wondered what it felt like to be cold-blooded. It seemed to her a terrible fate, a cosmic shunning. A kind of stark and absolute apartness, like floating in outer space. Not to be able to warm oneself or another. Touch made no difference in such a life. No-frills survival, Mary thought, drifting to sleep. No one expects a thing from him and he expects nothing in return, his existence singular and detached. There was true but abominable peace in such a thought. She imagined that she felt the dark weight of sleep settle on her, encase her protectively like a strange new skin.

The days prior to Christmas were long and shrill with cold. She'd dropped out of school fall semester and wouldn't begin at Catholic Academy until mid-January. Occasionally her friends Lisa and Bev dropped by to visit, but she refused to go out with them to places like McDonald's or down to the Rexall for a smoke—they were still sneaking *cigarettes!*

Once her dad invited her to lunch and she went. She wouldn't be seen by old high school acquaintances midday at the Steak & Ale. With her father she felt safe and, in an embarrassed way, womanly. She'd had a baby, after all, and he was her father who knew it. There seemed so many silences to fill that sometimes she dropped her fork on purpose, just to make a sound, just to have something to do. Three mornings a week she baby-sat so that Alexia could go to aerobics classes at the Y. Eke and her older brother, Brucie, attended school, so her only charge was Spencer, the baby.

Spencer was two and into everything, but Mary enjoyed his busyness. She made clay for him out of salt and dough, and they built simple things: totem poles and rainbow-colored snakes. On sunny days they trooped down to the barren winter park and collected sycamore balls, acorn crowns, rocks with mica, bottle caps. Once in a while they baked cookies. Sometimes she'd turn on "Sesame Street" and leave Spencer to his own devices. Then she'd go upstairs and feed Lord Alien mealworms, talk to him the way she might have written in a diary. Sometimes, and she knew this was crazy, she felt they understood one another. But then, just thinking of him that way, like a confidante, made her shake her head and laugh. Had she really gone backwards to this: such girlish safety and goodness?

Bev and Lisa bored her. They wanted to be friends with her, she could tell, and they tried hard. But she suspected that they only tried out of pity or out of an obligation to protect her from being a total outcast. They thought that she'd have nobody were it not for them.

Their sympathy, vast and ready, was ultimately self-serving. They tried to be her friends because they were curious. *Who was she now?* She was different and remote and her knowledge was forbidding.

Once, while Spencer was watching television, she imagined she was his mother, home alone with him all day while Jim Davenport worked. She planned to make spaghetti for supper and a chocolate pie. She planned to dress up, to bathe the baby and dress him in a fresh outfit before Jim came home. They'd be waiting at the door for him. All of them would eat dinner by candlelight and listen to soft music on the radio, and she and Jim would lean across the table, while the baby smiled at them, and kiss this glorious victory kiss. She held up her skirt in front of Eke's dresser mirror and gazed at the scar that spanned her pelvis. Then, she called Jim Davenport's number, but when his mother answered she hung up.

She tried to befriend her mother. Near Christmas they went shopping together. Her mother drank three cocktails at lunch and started crying in the lingerie department of Thalhimer's when Mary suggested that they buy a gift for the pregnancy counselor.

She tried to discuss their mother with Alexia, but Alexia defended her. "Look," she said, "it all makes perfect sense. Mom's miserable towards Daddy because he left. She's miserable towards me because I was their big mistake. She's miserable about you because you remind her of everything she threw away when she was seventeen. No wonder she sulks and tries to anesthetize herself. Look what a price she's had to pay for a few seconds of pleasure back in 1957. Except it's not really pleasure when you're so young," Alexia said grimly. "It's something else, but I sure wouldn't call it pleasure." She lit a cigarette and blew the smoke out through her nose.

"You think if Bruce left me, I'd act any different from Mother? Be any less miserable? Hell, I'd be *more* miserable, honey, because I'd be in jail. I'd have shot the bum."

When Eke got home from school, she begged Mary to take her to the Natural Science Center to see a special exhibition of reptiles. They took Alexia's Honda, and Eke played a tape by her latest favorite band, a British punk group called Edible Body Parts. Listening to the lyrics made Mary feel old: the arbitrariness of meaning, the aimless, chaotic rhythm. The music sounded goading and hostile, victimizing music like *na-nana-na-na* chanted cruelly out school bus windows. Mary imagined the band members spitting on an audience of cowering, tattered orphans. When she glanced at Eke, Eke was snapping her fingers to the beat, glassy-eyed.

It occurred to her that Eke might be experimenting with drugs. Mary had watched Alexia and Bruce roll a joint now and then, but they were always discreet. She wondered if Eke were happy. She wondered why every little girl she'd ever known, herself included, tried to rush life. She wanted to say: Don't do it, and her hand shot involuntarily from the steering wheel and closed over Eke's, squeezing it. Eke's hand was small and warm and dry, the stubby fingernails painted tomato red. It was difficult to imagine such a hand holding pills, a joint, an anole all in the same day. But Mary knew anything could happen nowadays and usually did.

"I knew you'd dig this group," Eke said, squeezing Mary's hand back. She closed her eyes and miraculously mouthed the nonsensical lyrics.

At the Natural Science Center they watched the feeding of the boa constrictors. A handsome young man offered the boas live mice. He talked a kind of lullabye talk to the snakes as he handled them. He called them names like Adam and Eve, and the audience laughed. He had strong, brown, sinewy arms. He wore a Hawaiian-style shirt printed with tigers and palm trees; the shirt made him seem exotic. Mary watched the young man entangle his arms with snakes until she felt she couldn't breathe, it was all so beautifully ghastly.

Once the young man smiled directly at Mary. He had a brown beard and kind brown eyes, and the smile should not have mattered, should have seemed the throwaway sort. Except that the young man's gaze lingered and appraised with an eagerness she hadn't earned. She left the room and went to the ladies' lounge and, inexplicably, washed her hands. She tried to summon a memory of her child. She took a brown paper towel and wrote "Christabel" in lipstick, folded it, and stuck it down inside her brassiere. Just let him try something funny, she thought. Just let him try.

Outside the bathroom, near the rocks and minerals display, she saw Eke, talking to a boy, holding hands. The boy was taller than Eke with longer hair and a bracelet. If she'd had a bad dream she could not have dreamed up worse. "I'm going," she said curtly. *"Now."*

Eke dropped her friend's hand and scurried after her. "Where'd you go? I looked everywhere."

But Mary didn't answer. "Who was that boy, Eke?" she cried as they buckled their seat belts. "Level with me. What in the hell are you up to?"

Eke looked at her as if she were crazy. "What are you talking about?" she said, incredulous. "That's my friend Angelica."

"Yeah, tell me another one," Mary said. "I know them all."

"What is this, the Inquisition?"

"Yes!" Mary shouted, slamming on brakes. "At the rate you're going, you'll be pregnant at eleven." She laughed bitterly. "Pregnant and foxy."

"You're weird and you're freaking me," Eke said, unbuckling her belt. "I'm getting out."

Mary lay her cheek against the steering wheel and began to cry. "Please don't get out, Eke," she said over and over. "Don't leave me."

"Okay," Eke said, touching her shoulder. "Just please stop acting like Mother for a while."

They drove on for several blocks in silence. "Maybe I need glasses," Mary said. "I mean if I thought Angelica was a boy."

"She's no boy," Eke sneered. "What an insult. Can we stop talking about her now, please?"

"I'm sorry, Eke," Mary said. "Sometimes I just forget."

"Forget?"

"Forget that you hate boys," Mary said.

"I hate the veritable guts of all boys," Eke said.

Mary smiled. She began to understand just how far she had traveled from innocence. When was the last time she had held a girlfriend's hand in public, swinging it, believing that touch was the most honest language of friendship?

The day before Christmas Eve she saw Jim Davenport. She was in the park with Spencer, playing hide-and-seek among the beech trees. Up the hill, on the opposite side of the park, she saw Jim Davenport walking with a girl. Most likely it was one of his sisters, but she couldn't tell. All the Davenports were tall, and this girl was as tall and slim and dark-haired as Jim. They wore shirts of similar plaid and they weren't holding hands. Mary's heart began to pound, but she was certain nobody could recognize her from such a distance. To them she was just some little tot's mother, out for a morning baby walk.

It was the way Jim Davenport walked that disquieted her; his kicking a can or a rock up the hill with each pace, a walk with a kind of disengaged energy. He hadn't been changed by any of it, had he? Still performing that glib, wasteful stride of energy without purpose that everybody young performed. The walk reminded her of the way he'd moved against her, planting her flesh with the hard sapling force of himself. In his hands she'd parted easily like soft earth.

Back at Alexia's she tried not to think of the way he'd kicked the can up the hill, his lean, tight, vigorous thigh. Alexia called and asked if she might go out to lunch with a friend, so Mary made sandwiches for herself and Spencer, then she put him down for a nap. She leafed through a *Good Housekeeping* filled with Christmas recipes, crafts, and fashions. She wanted Christmas to be over and January to arrive with piles of snow and people so bundled up that you couldn't recognize them, couldn't determine the shape of their bodies, male or female. Maybe she'd cut her hair short like Eke's and wear no lipstick like Angelica.

She went to the refrigerator and took out a couple of mealworms. She felt sorry for them in a way. Taken from their limbo of cold storage, they came alive gradually, seduced into activity by the heat of her hand. Awakened only to be devoured.

But the anole wouldn't eat. From beneath the slab of bark his eyes glinted dully. She put his cage under Eke's study lamp to warm him, but he flattened his head and closed his eyes. She dropped in a worm anyway, but he ignored it and slept. She watched him sleep. She imagined herself shrunken to his size, sleeping beside him. She wondered if it would matter, if her presence would be more comfort or burden. If only his lips were not so set. If only his face moved in recognition of her or his eyes lightened. It was his sameness that seemed merciless.

When Alexia got home, Mary was crying. She couldn't tell her why she was crying because Alexia would think she'd flipped out. A pathetic incommunicado lizard was dying, that's all. He was dying absolutely alone, lost in the outer space of himself. Why did she want him to feel otherwise?

Alexia held her for a while and rubbed her back. "It's probably just now hitting you, like a death," Alexia said. And Mary cried all the harder for Alexia's incomprehension. What was wrong with her that she'd never cried so hard about losing her baby? Somewhere deep

··· THE PAINFUL PARTS   171

within her she was dead to it all. She pretended otherwise to the adults in her life, but it had never been very real to her, the baby. She struggled from Alexia's embrace because she didn't deserve it. Alexia smelled of another life—restaurant spices, perfume. She was wearing little silver wishbone earrings.

"What nobody ever tells you, growing up, is that it's going to be one damn thing after another, plus MasterCard debt up to your eyebrows," she said. "A baby you didn't plan, a man you shouldn't have married, an unhappy love affair." She looked away quickly and lit a cigarette. "I ought to write a song," she said. She drew deeply on the cigarette. "Don't ever tell."

Mary felt confused, uncertain what her sister meant. She felt a heaviness in her chest, truth seeming to beat her from within like something trapped against its will. She wanted to touch the truth like she'd wanted to touch her baby, but she felt shy and out of place. The truth felt too soon for who she was. It had an aura like a flower picked from someone else's garden.

"Don't ever tell what?" she asked.

Alexia laughed, but without humor. "About *life*. It can be your revenge on the innocent. They have it too easy."

"Too easy?"

"Never mind," Alexia said briskly. "I keep forgetting you're just sixteen. *Sixteen*." She said "just sixteen" with a gift-giving exuberance. But when she repeated the word, she lingered over it as if trying to figure out how she could keep the gift for herself.

Eke and Brucie had gone to visit their Grandmother Ethyl in the mountains and wouldn't be back until tomorrow, Christmas Eve. Mary missed Eke. If Eke were there, she'd know what to do about Lord Alien, and Mary thought of calling her long-distance.

"He's been acting that way for days," Alexia said tiredly, flipping through her *60-Minute Gourmet* cookbook. "Frankly, I wish he'd go ahead and die. I hate keeping live worms in the refrigerator." She slammed the cookbook shut and said, "Let's all go to McDonald's tonight for supper."

Mary winced. "I don't want to go to McDonald's. It's so . . . public."

"So's life," Alexia said, "if you're to be any good at it."

On Christmas Eve afternoon Mary called the Natural Science Center to inquire about anoles.

"You'll have to speak with Mr. Morrison, our naturalist," the secretary said. "Hold, please." Mary listened for a while to a simpering recording of "Love, Love Me, Do." At last the secretary returned to say that Mr. Morrison had gone home early. After all, it was Christmas Eve. "But we'll be open December twenty-sixth," the secretary added brightly. "Happy holidays."

"Excuse me," Mary said, her voice resonant and forthright. "This may be a matter of . . . life and death."

There was a pause. "May I ask who's calling, please?"

"Oh, I don't know Mr. Morrison, if that's what you mean," Mary said. "I'm calling about a very sick animal."

"What kind of animal?" She sounded relieved. "Maybe someone else could help you."

When Mary told her it was an anole, the secretary admitted that anoles were Mr. Morrison's specialty. She took down Mary's name and number and promised to contact Mr. Morrison. "I'll have him call you just as soon as he can."

All afternoon, even through dinner, Mary crouched by the telephone biting her fingernails the way she used to while she waited for Jim Davenport to call. Eke came home and told her she was acting insane, but Eke had been grandmothered to death by Ethyl and was in a bad mood. "Let him die if he wants to," she said sullenly. "He knows what he's doing. Next time I'm getting a hermit crab, and I'm naming her Ethyl."

Alexia called everybody to come string popcorn for the Christmas tree, but Mary sat solemnly by the phone. She wasn't thinking about the anole anymore—this was the curious part. She'd begun to think wholeheartedly of Mr. Morrison.

Which one was he? She'd visited the Natural Science Center many times, strolling through the glittering displays of rocks and minerals, saltwater fish in shallow tanks, dinosaur bones, space technology. There were several friendly young men who worked there, eager to be asked questions, eager to show off their knowledge, their bravado. They could hold tarantulas without flinching, pressure an alligator's jaws into opening. They gathered up the snakes like jump ropes.

Was Mr. Morrison the man with the coiled brown muscles ready to spring from his tropical jungle shirt? The man with the soft-looking brown beard and eyes that had sorted through the crowd to smile at Mary?

Downstairs she could hear Alexia and her family singing carols, pulling it off: love and dissatisfaction co-existing. Love and grief. Love and loss. Even her mother was downstairs singing—what a miracle!

She imagined the phone ringing and Mr. Morrison speaking to her. She would describe the Lord in great detail, only certainly she would have to call him something else. She would posit theories: Was he depressed? Would he be happier with a mate? She heard herself laughing into the phone, yet telling Mr. Morrison: *"Don't* laugh."

And what if something should come of it? What if they continued talking, she and Mr. Morrison, and he was only a little older and they liked each other? What if she followed his expert advice and the anole got well? What if he called her back to check and she said yes, happy and grateful, and he was flattered and asked her out? Would she wear lipstick? What if he invited her to become his assistant at the Natural Science Center? What if her job was to hand him the mice to feed to the boa constrictors? Well, she would just have to be brave, wouldn't she? That was part of the deal.

Waiting for the phone to ring, a kind of greed rose up in her and she acknowledged it, indulged it, her hand poised over the telephone, poised to receive. Wouldn't she feel the ringing first in her bones, her skin humming with its summons as if touched? Listening, she could feel herself brightening into the hopeful girl she could not for the life of her resist.

oo oo oo

LYN LIFSHIN

The Daughter I Don't Have _____

jolts up in the middle
of the night
to curl closer than
skin, pink tongued
in a flannel dress
I wore once in some
story. I part her
hair braid her
to me as if to
keep what I can't
close, like hair wreathes
under glass in New
England or maybe
pull the hair into
a twist above the
nape of her neck,
kiss what's exposed
so wildly part of
me stays with her.
The child we will
not have is all
we wanted, all that
holds us together

JOYCE CAROL OATES

A Touch of the Flu _____

For years she tried to conceive a child, and failed; and failed at the marriage too—though "failed" is probably the wrong word, since, wanting a child so badly, and, as some observers (including her husband) said, so irrationally, she simply decided to give up on that man, and move on to another. And so she did; and conceived within months; and had her baby, a little girl; and lived with her alone, since, by that time, she'd come to understand that there was no room in her life for both the baby and the baby's father. Even had he wanted to marry her, which was not so clearly the case.

And she was happy with her little girl, if not, as she'd anticipated, ecstatic; except of course in bursts of feeling; wayward, unexpected, dazzling, and brief. These are the moments for which we live, she thought. She wondered if anyone had had that thought before her.

That summer she brought her daughter to Maine, to her parents' summer home, and there, each morning, pushed her in a stroller along the beach. She sang to her little girl, talked to her almost continuously, for there was no one in the world except the two of them, and, by way of the two of them, their delicious union, the world became new, newly created. She held her little girl in her arms, aloft, in triumph, her heart swelling with love, exaltation, greed. Sand, ocean, butterfly, cloud, sky, do you see? Wind, sun,—do you feel?

But one day she was overcome by a sensation of lightheadedness, and exhaustion, and returned to the house after only a few minutes on the beach, and handed the baby over to her mother, and went to bed; and did not get up for ten days; during which time she did not sleep, nor was she fully awake; simply lying in bed, in her old girlhood bed, her eyes closed, or, if open, staring at the ceiling, sightless and unjudging. Her mother brought her little girl to nurse, and she pushed her away, in revulsion, and could not explain; for it was herself she saw, in her mother's arms, as it had been, so suddenly, herself she'd seen, in her little girl, that morning on the beach; and she thought, I cannot bear it. Not again.

Still, the spell lifted, as such spells do. And she got up, and was herself again, or nearly; and nursed her baby again, with as much pleasure as before; or nearly. Her mother looked at her hard and said, "You've had a touch of the flu," and she smiled, and regarded her mother with calm wide intelligent eyes, and said, "Yes, I think that was it. A touch of the flu." And they never spoke of it again.

oo oo oo

DEA TRIER MØRCH

from: *Winter's Child* _____

The night nurse pokes at her gray head with her knitting needle.

"I could tell you about a woman who had nine miscarriages. Yes, nine! The tenth time she came in here and was in bed for eight and a half months."

"But didn't she have a flabby, weak baby?"

"No, not at all. It doesn't affect the children. She had the prettiest little girl imaginable. See for yourself. That's her, there."

She pokes with her knitting needle at a color photograph on the notice board. The photo is of a large round infant with a rattle in its hand, and with *Happy Christmas* underneath it in professional photographer's lettering.

"That was her firstborn. She was forty then. That's how strong the desire to have children can be."

The night nurse smiles.

"And you know what . . . a month ago, she had a boy. What do you say to *that*."

"She must have a good husband."

"Yes, she has! He's an engine-driver, and is totally involved in it all, otherwise it wouldn't have worked."

Marie looks round, feeling guilty that she is taking up the night nurse's time, but at the same time, it's nice to talk, so she plucks up her courage and goes on:

"But it's awful, isn't it, when you think about what women used to have to go through? When you think of the suffering involved in pregnancy and birth . . . the price they had to pay, and *still* have to pay, I suppose?"

"You *could* say that, when you see some of the women who come here. But don't forget this is a special department, my dear. Generally speaking, pregnancy has nothing to do with illness at all."

"But I can't help thinking about all those women who die in childbirth, or whose whole lives are ruined by it. Or those who've seen their babies die. Does anyone ever consider what great burdens they've borne?"

The night nurse looks sharply at her, like a bird, her head to one side.

"And what about pregnancy outside the womb?" Marie goes on. "And the fetus lying crookedly, and being strangled by the cord, and . . ."

Marie stares in front of her, her eyes wide.

"And birth cramps and rhesus negative ... and German measles ... and cleft palate and clubfoot and oxygen shortage and ...! Why is pregnancy such a frail affair? Why are the risks involved always played down ... at all levels ... so much? What's the reason for that? *That's* what I can't understand."

The night nurse turns up her transistor radio.

"Now just you come down to earth, will you? You're thinking too much about such things. Even here in this department, where the most difficult cases are, about *ninety-seven percent* of births are normal!"

Thank goodness the night is soon over.

· · ·

"You know, lots of Anders's workmates who have been present at their children's births don't want to sleep with their wives any more."

"You can't mean that!" exclaims Signe.

"Yes, they say they've had enough!"

Tenna scrapes her plate clean.

"How shitty of them, but that really can't be common," says Marie. "That means they regard their wives as ... well, as a kind of sex object."

"But Anders and I've never had a problem. We can't look at each other without...."

"How old are you?"

"Twenty-two, and he's just twenty-two, as well."

Tenna looks at Marie with her calm gray-blue eyes, then a spasm flashes across her face.

"Oh, hell...."

She drops her knife.

"There's something or other darned wrong," she says with tears in her eyes. "I'm oozing and I've still five weeks to go."

She pulls the cord above her head.

The nurse opens the door.

"Could I have a bedpan, please?" says Tenna.

Signe starts gathering up the crocks.

She picks up the tray and opens the door with one elbow.

Marie gets a woman's magazine off the window sill.

She opens it up and is soon gripped:

She felt two brutal arms around her. In one crazy moment, he again became a man. He was no longer ashamed and forced her to submit. He crushed her mouth down with a demanding kiss. Melting with gratitude, she let him undress her and with his large hands, he burrowed his way through to her naked flesh. Even before he had taken off her clothes, he was on top of her, forcing on her. . . .

"Finished," says Tenna to the nurse.

She puts a cloth over the bedpan and leaves the room.

. . . forcing on her his weight, his desire and movements. A sudden cramp made him rigid, motionless. When she half-opened her eyes, she saw Pierre's face crumple into an expression of ecstatic pain. Waves of desire continued inside her, then faded away, transformed into a need for tenderness and protection. . . .

Marie felt a kick inside her . . . *he crushed her mouth with a demanding kiss . . . ?*—now the child was off swimming again.

When Signe is back in her own ward, she goes on thinking about what they had talked about in Ward o, the things all patients in Prenatal think about incessantly.

About their sex life in relation to birth. About *vita sexualis*, as it is called in medical language.

Immediately after her first child was born, she found herself shaven, maltreated, torn, flayed, and sewn up! She had felt slayed. She had not thought reality would be as harsh as that.

For weeks she had been frightened even to bend down and look at her swollen and patched sexual parts. Not until a month later, when her body had calmed down, did she dare look at herself down there in a mirror she had put on the floor.

She had wondered whether they would ever sleep together again. The constant flow of fluids from pregnancy, the newborn infant at her breast, the endless exhaustion. Everything seemed to put obstacles in the way.

Neither men nor women really know anything about a woman's vagina. A dark and mysterious place, as puzzling as the starry sky. The work of the gynecologist and the astrologist are both equally far from the ordinary mortal's understanding.

But childbirth throws its merciless light on a woman's sexual organs. The vagina is revealed and demystified, and if either partner's sexual life has been exclusively based on this mystification, it is bound to fall to pieces. Naturally.

That was probably why Anders' friends that Tenna had mentioned no longer wished to sleep with their wives, after they had seen for the first time the raw mincemeat between her legs. The pinup girls of the newspapers and then a real live birth . . . they don't really go together.

Signe has talked to Jacob about whether he was scared about their sex life when he had seen his first child born.

"No, not at all," he had answered in surprise. "I don't really connect the two things, birth and sex. Do you? Sex life has nothing much to do with the sexual organs. You mustn't think that. It's to do with relations between two people."

Remarkably enough, they had started to sleep together again, even more relaxed, pleasantly, and simply than before, if not quite so frequently, because of the children.

And yet a great deal has changed. Sexuality is no longer so much self-knowledge. Not so self-centered. And not so essential.

. . .

But no, it is an ordinary weekday in the department for newborn babies. No alchemy, no mystique connected with it. That forest . . . is the cables, cords, tubes and drips casting their shadows up on to the walls and ceiling.

The children in the incubators are those who have been ejected too early from the mother organism, either because it was not in a state to retain them any longer, or because the climate in there had suddenly become too harsh.

Others have at the very last moment been released from the body's stranglehold via a Caesarian.

Some of them are even below 1,000 grams in weight . . . the weight that is otherwise the borderline between miscarriage and newborn.

There they lie . . . Winter's Children . . . in their mechanical wombs of glass and steel, condemned to survive.

Red and green or transparent tubes carry nourishment through their nostrils down into their stomachs or through their skin into the bloodstream.

They are children born too early, and children with a fault somewhere, children with visible or invisible inborn defects, children for whom some complication has arisen during or after their actual birth.

One of them has meningitis and a far too pale pink skin. Another has faulty heart valves and is apt to turn the color of bilberries. One has a broken arm from a complicated Caesarian birth. And there . . . a drug addict on a cure.

Some of them are having blood transfusions. Some lie in respirators. Others are receiving oxygen or lie immobile in sharp light, their eyes bandaged. Some tremble. Some have drawn breath in the womb.

A new patient is carried in, an absolutely new baby brought into the world a moment ago, its life hanging on a thread. The first day is the most critical in a human being's life. More people die during the very first day than during any other day in their existence.

"Little Lukas's father is on the phone."

"Oh God, what shall I say to him?"

"Tell him the truth."

The young doctors are sitting on high stools, observing their patients through glass walls. They talk, gesticulate, and laugh.

They listen to the news on the radio, which can be heard faintly in the background.

A nurse is carefully carrying a little surgical patient. His head is swollen. He resembles a monster, a monster of the kind you read about in ghost stories. They have wound a white bandage round his neck; his tongue sticks out, stiff and thick between blood-red lips, bubbles coming from the corners of his mouth.

She carries him round between the incubators, kissing his pale little hand, and looking down into his gentle eyes. They are clear and look straight back at her. He is not newborn. He has been there a couple of weeks and has already had several operations.

She whispers something to him and he turns his heavy little head toward the sound. He tries to smile, but the smile is nothing but a twitching round his eyes. She sees it at once and smiles back.

He has been baptized long ago. He has his own independent first name. Most of these children have ... large, solid adult names betraying the dreams and hopes of their parents.

No trouble is spared to ensure their survival, to get them to cope with life as well as possible. No treatment is too demanding or too expensive.

This country is a closed country. No unauthorized person is let in.

But if, like Marie, you happen to see it ... if only through a glass pane in a door, then you cannot help thinking about how dearly bought life is, how beautiful it is. And how cruel it is.

—translated by Joan Tate

oo oo oo

CAROL BERGÉ

from: *Acts of Love: An American Novel* _____

Ellen was pregnant. She knew it from the third day after she conceived. She was totally familiar with her body. Her breasts swelled and were tender. When she took off her bra at the end of the day, the breasts swung forward and there was real pain, especially near the glands up under the arm. Not like any other body response, and she recognized it, although she had never experienced it before. She was startled; she *knew*.

She waited until she was a week late for her period; by then, she was almost two weeks certain. It was the tiny but strong and different womb-sensations around the time that her period would have been due, and the absence of the usual pre-menstrual cramps: no temperament shifts, and no small and then wide cramps. The slight nausea and the feeling of intense hunger between meals. She knew and knew, twenty times a day.

"Love is so dangerous," she thought. She saw Edward, said nothing to him, looked at his vaccination mark, tried to visualize what he had looked like as a baby. He had pictures of his own boys as babies; the oldest looked just like Kathy (thereby confirming the Edwardian theory of genetics), or what Kathy had once looked like; the big bones were there and the coloring and shape of face, but not the overlay of misery-fat Kathy had added. His younger boy looked more like Edward. But then, Ellen was thinking, what if I had a boy—he would look more like me than like Edward, and no one would know he was the father except me. And, *if* he wanted to know, Edward . . .

Maybe she would not tell Edward; she thought he would panic: he was now, over a year after Kathy had left, still in the pain of that mess with her. And, of course, he was seeing Myra. A lot. Ellen sat at the kitchen window every morning, looking out at the field in a manner that was parallel to the way her twin looked at and into and past the brown wall of the barn from that other window. And no answers came . . .

She wanted a baby. This baby. Edward's. But really hers—she couldn't count on anyone else, she would have to assume that Edward, if he knew, might move away from the closeness with her . . . she could not think much or deeply about this: touched it, veered away, came back to it. Could she decide to have the baby and to raise it alone. When she couldn't even take full-time care of the colt! But what else was there to do. *Not* have it? Not possible!

She went over to Frey one day. Just to be around her and to try to let the feelings sift out toward some answer. Frey gave Ellen no answers. Said things that Ellen already knew; that she knew Ellen already knew; things designed to keep Ellen open to the possibilities: "Whenever a woman conceives, there's a reason; no woman ever conceived 'by accident' ..." and then, "Humans are so different from animals, even though they're animals; they're instinctive, but they don't have the sense to organize it for themselves and realize they're a lot more than that—they convince themselves that things happen to them by chance, when they could finally realize that they do things like conceiving for a reason, something more than propagating the species, a damn important reason or two ..."

As they walked around the farm, talking, Frey doing some chores, Ellen helping or just being there, Ellen was thinking, "flashing," as Edward called it, the small insights coming with Frey's comments. Turning things over. True: she must recognize that she was glad to conceive because it would give her a bond to Edward—in the timeless way of woman to man. And it would be a way to force him to recognize her love for him and the direction of it, and her own feeling of wishing to feel bound to him. In this she felt blameless: it seemed a classic gesture. But would he recoil. Having had two children by Kathy. With his particular history, he would probably ultimately recoil and run, in despair at the entrapment. So she would be faced with having the child alone, and keeping it alone, and raising it alone.

The strong possibility of an abortion. The death idea again. And Frey, saying, "When you kill another living thing, you are killing a part of yourself—but then there's that other side of it, a death gives more available energy to what is already alive on earth," and, later, "An early thaw sometimes means a longer season of growth, but then, a late thaw sometimes means a more intense shorter season ..." and all of this Ellen took in and took away with her.

The ideas and feelings sifted slowly as she moved through her days. She would not tell Edward. She would assume total responsibility for what would be occurring within her own body. She would realize and face the reality—that Edward would not say, "Hey, that's *great*," or, "Let's keep the baby and raise it together," he would never say what she thought she wanted to hear from him. If Edward was who she loved right now, the idea of the baby would estrange him from her. And if she told him and he said *No*, she would feel bitterness; now, she did not feel bitter toward him or toward herself.

She worked in her garden. Noticing the pine seedlings that grew randomly near the tidy cultivated rows of her plantings. Each of them a strong little tree, a tiny well-formed tree. And when she drove past the Reservoir, there were the intentional plantings of pine trees, in which the rows were only clearly noticeable from certain angles, like parts in hair. An intentional forest, to enrich the land: thinned out scientifically: a planned forest, dense, the needles as heavy at their base as if they were not told where to fall.

She thought too about a photograph she had, of a sculpture made of four paintings and two plaques and a box: the sections were called, and the piece was titled, "A Birth/A Bird/A Man/A God/A Love/A Death" and it was torn out of a newspaper's art section and taped to her wall in the kitchen near her stove. Where she could glance at it, get into it, and ponder on it ... And thought about what Edward had told her about his brother Levon: who had married and had two sons, but found out (or knew?) that neither of the boys was his; one of them was the child of his closest friend, Duane Rattermann, and the other, he never did find out about. He had already formed his emotional attachment to the boys by the time he found out, and the marriage was going to continue. The delicate thralls, the binds, tapes, webs between people. Levon Richthoven wanted his wife anyhow; the wife wanted the marriage, the boys, and, somehow, in her own peculiar way, Levon ... Edward thought the whole thing was a mess and said so, from his righteous Capricorn conventionality, and said he was beyond trying to figure out anyone else's motivations, let alone his own—nothing seemed reasonable or predictable. For their part, Levon and his wife had made their peace. They said nobody could write the rules for *them*! Ellen liked them for that.

Finally, in one instant of desire, she decided to have an abortion. And the minute she decided, she acted on the decision. Then there was time to react to having made the decision. She thought about what Myra might say if she knew Ellen was pregnant by Edward. Myra!— would surely never allow herself to get pregnant—and Ellen laughed at herself, realizing the edge to that: her thinking of it that way confirmed what Frey had said, about every woman knowing damn well what she was doing when she got pregnant; Ellen had indeed "allowed" herself to get pregnant.

Ah, but she missed the baby already, having made that crisp decision. There was a hunger in her arms to hold a baby. And it was the destruction of a life—a life that was part Ellen and part Edward and totally itself. This idea brutalized her and she could not dismiss it. She had not been raised Catholic and it was not a question of ethic. But she was Pisces. She had to decide she could not afford such maunderings. It was just not *practical* to have this child at this time. Maybe there would be another child, another time; maybe not. Aaah, what if there were no other time, no other baby for her ... to hold, to raise, to love ... She had to hold back those feelings, those thoughts which threatened to change her from determination to emotionality.

The field she worked in was a reminder that there was this season, and the one before, and the one ahead—and the years. Perhaps there would be another chance for her to have a child. Earth takes care of its own. She felt she should go ahead now. Before she changed her mind. She called to make an appointment with a doctor in the City. Even from within the clarity of the decision, she felt the deep twinge of misery and resentment at having to go through with this. She arranged to take three days away from her work and went into the City to the metropolitan hospital. Superficially, the abortion went without complications; she was, as the doctor confirmed, wondrously healthy, and could expect a fast and uneventful recovery, and would find no problems were she to conceive again at a future time . . .

It was on the trip back from the City that the depression of the event hit her. She sat on the train and wept. She missed the child that had left her body, she felt bereft as after a death of someone one had known. She ached for it, she wanted to hold it, she knew she was not being reasonable; but then, was life reasonable? Wasn't it just as reasonable, as healthy, as life-confirming to *want* that baby, to want to raise that child; to want to confirm her place on earth as a woman by having that baby? She wept . . .

She wept. Mourned. And when she was done, she had mourned in a way that resembled her keening at Tom's sudden death. Part of the mourning was done now. There was no way to cope with either death. She would mourn now, as she had done then, and she would have to manage to be enough of a person to continue to move along within her own life despite the deaths. There would be no living separate from death. It was all of the same fabric. No way to separate the one from the other; it was not two substances, two states called "life" and "death"—it was *lifedeath*, it was a Winter that was also a Summer, a seed that was a tree that was finally back into earth again and a tree. She would live with this new pain as she had with the old. And time would change its texture as it had in the past. It was a reasonable pain; it came in waves, she thought she might learn to deal with it.

SUMMER BRENNER

Inches and Lives _____

Plant seeds about 1 inch deep. About 8 seeds per foot in a row.
Space rows 3 feet apart. Seeds germinate in 9 to 15 days. When seedlings are
2 inches tall, thin or transplant to 3 inches apart. Tie plants to trellis or support.
Needs non-acid rich soil with good drainage.

The yard in New Mexico was full of clay. Kaolin. And we had to get
sawdust and chicken manure. And work hard to get the ground ready.
Our friends helped a lot. It was to be a big garden. And everyone
would share the work and vegetables. Squash and chile and melons
grew easily. Radishes too. Suddenly one day we had hundreds of them.

Laura made a beautiful scarecrow with different colored ribbons and
lots of bells. Farmers said the best way to keep the crows off was to
kill one and hang it up in a tree. Then they'd all know they weren't
welcome. I was really fond of those little crows. And it was so curious
to me the way they too loved New Mexico and would stay there into
the winter. Especially in the cemetery near Albuquerque, you could see
them stuffed in the limbs of the big bare trees.

I suspected I was pregnant. My period was late. But that wasn't so
unusual. Paul and I had just come back from California. And traveling
has always confused my body. What really notified me was the way
everything smelled. Different. Precious and disgusting. Cilantro always
reminds me of that kind of smell.

It took them three minutes of stirring a small amount of my urine to
tell me the test was positive. Positively. I smiled and swallowed and
walked out. Walking out of anywhere in New Mexico was a shock.
The sun was always so bright. I kept blinking to try to get my heart
in focus.

Call Paul. I telephoned. No answer. Maybe he was at the bar. The
bar. The baby. The baby bar. The candy bar. The Baby Ruth. The
baseball bar. The baseball bat. The bat. The baby. Inside me. *Seeds*
germinate in 9 to 15 days.

I got in the car and drove up to Placitas. At least if Paul wasn't there,
I could go see Laura. Or Tom and Lonnie might be home. And Tom
was a doctor.

Oh God. What was the story he told me about the cameras with
microscopic needles. That they could inject needles anywhere in the
body and take pictures of what was happening. And that in abortions,
even very early ones, the limbs were already visible. And the sucking

machine just tore them off and whisked them away like tiny match-sticks.

Baby. Names. Boy. Girl. Darling. Tiny pussy cock. Family. Baby bunny. Peas. I'll have to get those peas in the ground this afternoon. *In rows 3 feet apart.*

And what would Paul say. I said I'd always be ready to have an abortion. Every woman's right. No more unwanted children in a world filled up with unwanted adults.

Unwanted. Wanted. Room. Womb. Bent up. She couldn't even feel that tiny bean. Buried somewhere in her rich female soil. Soiled and spoiled. A garden going to waste. They didn't want a baby. Her body already sowed and working. Not the right time. At least not for her. The garden. That was where she wanted to watch things grow. Out there under the stars.

She took a left off the highway and drove up the mountain. Paul was in the bar. She sat down and ordered a brandy.

"What's the celebration?"

Annie didn't say a word.

When seedlings are 2 inches tall. Paul I'm pregnant. I'm pregnant Paul. Paul I'm going to have a baby. Paul we're going to have a baby Paul.

Paul looked at her steady profile. "What's wrong?"

"Well I just went to the doctor."

"You're pregnant!"

They got in the car to drive back home. Well honey I think that's great. Don't you. I mean don't you. It seems OK. Don't you. I mean it's fine with me. Don't you. Why don't you say something? Why don't you talk to me? It's great isn't it. You love kids. Don't you. Don't just sit there like the world just ended. Don't you. Scream. Kiss me. I think it's great. Annie. Annie.

"I've already made up my mind. I'm going to have an abortion."

They were kind. They were very kind. The nurse asked her if she wanted a pill. She lay down on the table. The pillows. The sheets. The stirrups. The small vacuum machine. The swooshing noise. The counting. God it really hurt. Like something being taken out of you that didn't want to go. Like the abalone content in its shell that didn't want to go. Like the inside of a walnut that has to be picked. Like mosses and cactus fruit. Like honey in combs. Tangles in hair. Something stubborn and content.

Her body beat and stung. All of her ached. Empty now. Clean now. Hollow again and ready now. O it's not so easy. *Tie plants to good drainage.*

oo oo oo

SUMMER BRENNER

Letter to an Unborn Daughter _____

November 18, 1976

My dear girl, I know there is very little I can say to you
That you don't already know. I can't help but think of
You as someone beautiful that I would be holding in my arms.
That my oldest child your brother would wonder about.
The softness and quickness you would have. And sure and steady
Eye you would hold us all with. Just like your father we'd say.
Just like his mother.
A deepness in brown like the forest.
A long trip to your heart. Though not slow or reluctant.
Say like tall trees. And what is called deep woods.
We would endure much to know you. Not in the sense that it would be
Difficult but the details would be overwhelming.
Fixtures of fur in your irises.
Where your brother would be obvious you would disappear.
I want so much of this, so much holding this perfect roundness
That it's very sad for me to send you back before we've even begun.
And I know this may be our one chance to know you like this.
You can see why I have regrets. The pain aside. And your wrench
Being the worst and the one I care about.
Your father is concerned. And seeks in his endearing way
To study better the forces in the universe.
I'm riding on the faith of my strings that it will be OK.
And that whatever it was you had to do here can be put off
Or transferred.
I'll never forget the magic of your presence. Really you're so gentle
And Lord knows we could use that after your brother's rampage.
He'll miss you a lot dear. We all will.
But I know you'll have a good night.

oo oo oo

LAURA CHESTER

from: *The Stone Baby* _____

The beating of her belly seemed to have transferred to a pounding in her head. The throb, the beat of blood, inside her, couldn't be picked up. The panic of their searching, under the surveillance of machines, slicked to the belly, recording what was nothing, that registered on the face of the nurse who probed, almost prodding, trying to find that heartbeat, but the sound wasn't there.

Kate read her face and knew.

The nurse looked down, ashamed. She said she'd get the doctor.

Kate said, "It's alright."

Conrad started to cry. His knowledge came with immediate tears, until wracked, shaking, and Kate held Conrad's hand and tried to comfort him. "It's going to be alright. It's really all o.k.," knowing now that the baby was dead, that it wasn't alive inside her, and yet she felt illuminated by some larger grace, some force that was moving through her, that still had to deliver her, and she felt the peace of it, the calm before the shock hits, unable to absorb what had actually happened inside her. The true impact of that would only come much later in much fuller force than anyone could feel right now, like a tidal wave, internal, to knock her down, to bash her down, to hold her there, under the churning blackened water, until she could hardly breathe, to hold her, pressing down with the force and weight of tonnage, as if she too should die, but that realization hadn't even dawned yet.

The doctor was in the room. His expression was like that of a basset hound, she thought, mournful, and yet amusing to her. His serious, clean hands. Everything about him seemed overly neat and tidy, and she wondered why doctors were so immaculate, when life was such a mess. She shut her eyes and pictured him with a shining, silver spade, standing on the top of a garbage heap, gulls whirling overhead, making gull jokes about him, as if he could find anything worth keeping here, on this heap of rubbish, in his expensive, clean, pressed clothes.

But now his hands were in her, testing. The chill of the iron, the smooth cool silvery parts of the bed, the rails, she hung onto, the tiny delicate wallpaper like some fine, fine emotion, some fragrance on the cheek of her grandmother, Baba, some buttercup of life, denial, crushed underfoot, the tiniest little flower, smashed, intentional, No—this couldn't be.

Conrad's face was streaked with grief. And the doctor took the stethescope from his ears, as if he'd heard enough of that music, and he was saying what was obvious, that their baby wasn't breathing. The perfect heart was silent. But still in there. Mild labor. And very large. An extremely large baby. But not born. And it still had to be born. The slow, powerless labor. They agreed on an injection. And he looked concerned about her. He looked at her oddly. But she didn't feel that she was the odd one. All of *them* were odd. Outside. Outside this fact, looking in at her, as if through the nursery glass, while she was in the eye, still, poised, perfectly at one, inside the eye of the cyclone, the funnel through which she'd pour. She held their baby in. It was hers, a part of her. But she was strong now. She would give it birth, give her baby birth, and then the medication took hold and the contractions became very real, and she was unable to think about anything else, but her hair seemed in the way, and she snapped at Conrad to DO something with her Damn Hair. "Pin It UP!" And then she told him to stand back. The energies were releasing the cool grey infant coming— pushed, as any other, pushed and pounding against the quickly dilated cervix, splitting her then, huge, the head, she felt it with her hand. So strange to feel that hardness, head, and then to feel the rest, inside her, coming—she moaned, again, the shoulders, the body being born, pulled up by the hands of the doctor in his rubber gloves, all greased, and the body was a slithering mass, with very real hair, dark brown, and she laughed, and then gulped as she saw, "A boy," and she reached down, completely herself without pain now, and the doctor, bless him, helped her hold the baby in her arms, before the placenta had even come, but on the next contraction it did, and he was so large, and healthy look-ing, perfect, "Conrad, look at his hands," and his toes, his feet, so perfect, "My God," and the nurse was standing there saying that it was time.

"Wait," she looked up at her husband, and said plainly, "Isn't he beautiful? The most beautiful, baby boy?" But this started Conrad crying again, bawling, almost like Atea she thought, so extreme, his anguish rising to the surface so quickly like their daughter. Kate had no need to cry, she thought. This baby was enough. But Conrad didn't want to hold the baby. He couldn't, but she wanted to. "Just one more minute."

The nurse waited with a cloth in her hands. They always wanted the mother to hold the baby, to know that this was something that had actually happened, that this was death, not life, that this was silence, not screaming, that this was actual, not breathing, but not to let her hold the child too long. "Alright now dear," the kind nurse said, for this time it was not a question. So quickly those attachments bind, so firmly they remain, fiercely bound, forever, as he already was, but she handed the baby over, and they wrapped him, and took him, and her eyes lunged after—how she had wanted that baby!

MILK SONGS

oo oo oo

SHARON OLDS

New Mother _____

A week after our child was born,
you cornered me in the spare room
and we sank down on the bed.
You kissed me and kissed me, my milk undid its
burning slip-knot through my nipples,
soaking my shirt. All week I had smelled of milk,
fresh milk, sour. I began to throb:
my sex had been torn easily as cloth by the
crown of her head, I'd been cut with a knife and
sewn, the stitches pulling at my skin—
and the first time you're broken, you don't know
you'll be healed again, better than before.
I lay in fear and blood and milk
while you kissed and kissed me, your lips hot and swollen
as a teen-age boy's, your sex dry and big,
all of you so tender, you hung over me,
over the nest of the stitches, over the
splitting and tearing, with the patience of someone who
finds a wounded animal in the woods
and stays with it, not leaving its side
until it is whole, until it can run again.

oo oo oo

NAOMI SHIHAB NYE

The Rattle of Wheels Toward the Rooms of the New Mothers ⸻

Down the hallways came the rolling alert, at midnight, four A.M., with the generous humming of nurses in doorways giving instruction, promising they'd be back. From those high hospital beds with special buttons for raising, lowering, those islands on which the tailbone ached and the startled breasts grew and grew, we heard the rattling as a boat coming to save us, the answer to our unshaped cry.

I wanted to hold the nurse in my arms too, she had all the information. How to negotiate the compact swaddled bundle, to connect rosebud lips with raw and blossoming nipple, to make it hold. Something like electricity. Tapping in to the source. But who was the source? Was he? Was I? Hold him like a football, they all said, and I did not think to say how little that helped.

What if he never ate? What if his elegant eyes stayed rapturously closed in on themselves and the silent world was all he needed? An elderly nurse, Specialist in Rousing Sluggish Babies, turned him upside down, tickled his feet. She advised me to be patient. A series of swirling TV lessons—"How a Newborn Perceives"—unfolded on the screen. I attended a bath demonstration where one veteran mother just brushing up on skills offered her fleshy redhaired daughter to be dipped and patted dry. I eavesdropped on a Bengali couple in the hall anguishing over names; whatever they had produced was the opposite of what they had prepared for. I could not apply the sticker to my door. "IT'S A BOY" which declared so much less than what I was feeling. It's an Angel, a Miracle—how easy, contagious, to reduce this miracle to sex and weight.

He was ... petite. They unwrapped him under a spotlight in the hospital nursery, took blood counts, he was wearing tiny blinders, soaking in the glow, barely flickering an arm or leg—"like some beachcomber," my husband whispered—and I stood at the nursery window watching him bask till I trembled and a nurse came to place her hands on my shoulders. She guided me toward the chamber of incubators. "Now *these*," she said, "These are worth trembling for, these are *really little*, but yours is simply yellowish. He's also slightly cold. He will be fine."

When the volunteer in striped hospital jumper came to sell me the portfolio of ugly "First Day Photos," I wept. What if he never made it out from under the light and these scrunched-up eyes and closed fists were all I took home? Relics, ancient sad baby stories, poking their fingers into fitful dreams. Beyond the hospital windows, heavy rain was sheeting down, sky booming and blackening repeatedly, it was the peculiar June of endless rain, streets flooded, the babies pressed to our sides.

I felt revived each time my husband came. It was possible to ask about our house and the world outside, to laugh together at another new father who pointed proudly through the nursery window, proclaiming to relatives, "Isn't the nose just like Cheryl's? And look at those hands, big as mine!"—then realized it wasn't his baby.

It was possible to laugh over our recent saga of birthing, how I'd sent him to the grocery for lemons, desperate for my old favorite Arabic dish of lentils and rice with lemony salad on top, and he'd returned to find me in bed, clutching my side, "Oh, oh, something's not right," never thinking *this was it*—later, in final throes of breathing and counting at hospital, I'd puffed to the labor nurse, "Are you *sure* this isn't a false alarm?" so she hooted and told every passing nurse what I'd said.

My husband and I walked the whole wing arm-in-arm, watching nurses swab the freshest babies, till a stricken cowboy, collapsed against a wall, noticed our eyes on him and blurted, "My baby didn't make it and my wife may not either"—changing the day. What could we bring this man? Coffee, juice? Why didn't the nurse take him in her arms too?

Into the swaths of clean linen, the stacked towels, I wept. Buried myself in a closet, weeping and weeping. Why had this crossroads pumped so many tears into my eyes, abundant wellsprings, like the endless dripping of the stone cave in Syria where I'd prayed for this baby, a craggy nun directing me to drink, drink from the pool at the bottom, fill my bucket—if a hundred people filled their buckets at once, the level would not go down, she said. And I'd drunk, praying. I'd also drunk water from Lourdes, swallowed herbs, rubbed the subtle essence of rosemary and melissa oils on my belly, leaning toward this moment with senses tuned toward babies, their closed and haloed eyes, their hallowed empty hearts.

One of the four nights at the hospital they forgot to bring him to me. I awakened fifteen minutes early, preparing myself, raising the bed, straightening the covers. Far off down the halls I could hear the parade of rattling begin and envisioned the little bundled worlds on wheels each heading toward a different door, mothers groggy and roused, some more anxious than others, and some more ecstatic. It was easy to notice the matter-of-factness of third- and fourth-time mothers; I'd heard their casual chatter as they hoisted the bundles, joking about diapers, saying, "Here we go again." And what about the 16-year-old down the hall, less than half my age, her bland face still unformed, her rocky vocabulary a smattering of Yeahs and Gees? It seemed preposterous that some people fell into this experience with no apparent forethought, while others struggled years to be here . . . maybe it was the same about everything in life.

Wheels rattling to halts at bedsides, the occasional yelp and cry, and the one baby whose long siren of a wail stitched all our rooms together.

I waited and waited and no wheels stopped at my door. Why hadn't I limped down the hall to collect him myself? Panic flashed—something had happened. He'd gone from chilly to frozen. He'd slipped away while I was sleeping and they hadn't told me. I pounded my call button till the drawl flooded my speaker, "Can I help you?"

"Where is my baby?" I called out. "The wheels are heading back to the nursery already and my baby never arrived!"

"We'll check."

The gap of centuries. The aching pit of longing. The terror of loss, now that he was finally here, and the whole lineage of mothers, bruised and troubled, echoing behind me . . . rosaried Mexican mothers keeping vigil at Our Sacred Heart, chanting stroking Arab mothers, the mothers of Calcutta stoking dung fires before their tumbled cardboard shacks . . . would faith follow the fear? Would wisdom come suddenly now? And bellowed the voice, "They just forgot to bring him. They gave him a bottle already and he went back to sleep. Do you need the breast pump?"

How I tumbled into dreams after that, hugging the fatly anonymous hospital pillow, dreaming the lips of babies, that sucking pull, the sigh and swallow, dreaming the nights ahead when each fine-tuned whimper would pull me back to earth, unfolding fists around a finger, dreaming the earth's secret rattle as it turned in space on its ancient implacable hinge.

oo oo oo

RACHEL HADAS

Up and Down _____

Days into weeks.
Still night sweats
and bleeding still,
its bleachy smell.
Your bleat softly
shears the thick
fleece of dark.
I wake wet,
cold, hot:
milk and sweat,
nightgown, hair,
humid breasts.
Here you are.
Latch on.
Suck.

Lie down, says the old body.
Get back between the sheets.
Root down, down in dreams.

Your soft call cries no more alternatives.
The bed, the night
make space for three of us.
Silent accommodations in the dark.

MARIE HARRIS

Milk _____

The goat comes to me nameless and sick, her udder swollen with the memory of her dead kid. I bring her hay and grain and water warmed against a March morning, pull the first yellow milk from under her until it whitens and spurts into the pail.

. . . My breasts are swollen. I don't know how. The baby is frantic and I cannot let go. I am crying. My son tastes salt in his milk, hears a new pulse, sucks.

Head at her flank, listening to her digestion move like unfamiliar scales, I milk her: thumb and forefinger circled at the top of the teat, sucking down with three fingers and palm. I squat in her stall, listening.

. . . he pushes at me. I give him more. He sings in his sleep.

After the last milk squirts into the pail, there is more. Nudge the udder. There is more and it is the sweetest and richest. Strip the milk out and the goat will give more next time. Strip her dry.

. . . Crying brings me out of sleep. Crying pulls me out of half-finished dreams. My milk is vinegar and hyssop.

It's early. I am milking a goat and looking at a maple red with spring.

It's early. I am nursing a baby under a gray window.

The letters of my name are spelled in milk. Milk is the perfume I wear. The letters of my name make a new constellation. I cannot set a course by any of its stars.

oo oo oo

ANNE WALDMAN

Sonne _____

Could
anything
mean more to me
right now
than the
boy's smile
as he turns
on belly
lifting his face—

his
muscles
get
stronger

he laughs
throwing his
head back
as I toss him
around my lap

and he wants
to put the purple iris
inside
his pink mouth

no no
no no no, nothing.

oo oo oo

JOYCE THOMPSON

Dreams of a New Mother _____

Birth is inconvenient, incomplete, unjust, an imperfect separation. Once you rode together through the nights and days, the flexing of her toes a tickle inside your ribs, her twists and squirms a mute communication, reassurance that you prospered jointly, your welfares utterly congruent. Now you are here and she is there. She sleeps and you do not. You listen to her sleep. The slightest of her sighs sets off sirens deep in your brain. You chase molecules across the ceiling, imaginary flecks of moving black, run the sheep backwards, toward wakefulness, forbid yourself to be seduced by the silent warmth of the husband who sleeps beside you, or lulled by the long, slow rhythm of his breaths. Sternly forbid yourself the pleasures of the deep, kind bed and smooth sheets, refuse to board the nightlong, headlong brain-vacation train that races by so fast it makes a wind that brushes your cheek in the dark. You must not, dare not board and ride, because your baby sleeps in her crib a million miles away across the room and must not wake to find you gone. Kinetically familiar, she is visually new, unimaginably small. Her needs are simple and immense. She was born holding your heart in her hands, clutching your nerves like reins in her tiny fists.

You must not dare not must not dare not must not dare not long to need to ache to absolutely must not dare not will not sleep.

The meat is red and raw, oozing beef blood, a large, crude roast you clutch in sticky hands. The boy tries to take it by force. Larger than you, he is still growing, devours everything in sight to fuel the last push into manhood. You fight bitterly, this bloody hunk of protein the prize. He wants it to grow, you need it to survive. All bonds are broken, all bets off. You are both beyond sharing. There is no love in your heart, and none in his eyes. He grabs your arm and twists it painfully behind you, while you kick and claw without restraint, trying to reimburse him pain for pain.

The baby cries. You wake and rise to feed her. Only her body wakes this time. Her eyelids are puckered shut and she sucks blindly at your breast.

You recant before the testimony of your senses. The house exists. The ruddy mantlepiece and gray-pink rug, the round pink ottoman whose rolling you rode as a child. Familiar scent of pomander, of dusty rose, old wool, false leather, burning wood, and walnut oil to make the baby grand piano shine. The china dog and burnished vase are safe upon their shelf. Your mother is not dead. If you can find her and apologize for the misapprehension of death, she will not die to you again. Your baby lives, and needs your milk to go on living. It is long and dangerously past her feeding time and she screams with hunger, somewhere out of sight. Two lives to save, and you must answer for two deaths, rooted here in sensuous memory, trapped between generations, unable to move.

The baby cries. You wake and rise to feed her. In the nest of her covers, with her thin neck and ruffled hair, she is a small bird, angry at her hunger. Crying. Until you feed her and she sleeps again.

The baby bites your nipple off and spits it out in the dusty corner behind your rocking chair. Blood pours from the wound, and you are paralyzed by hurt. The baby howls in rage at the red milk that flows so fast and tastes so salty strange until, infinitely adaptable, she rallies and learns to drink your blood.

The baby cries. You wake and rise to feed her. The sky has just begun to lighten behind the blind, and in the grainy bedroom light, you can see her one-eyed sideways blue stare above your breast, hunger even more intense than love.

She is lost through your fault, your own most grievous fault. You were living your life, in the midst of doing something that gave you minor pleasure, gossiping or talking politics, and you forgot, misplaced her. Where? It is hours since she ate. Your breasts are throbbingly full. The laughter of children leads you to a bedroom with a triptych mirror above the dresser, a mahogany bedstead dark and solemn as a grave. There on the bed, a small boy lies beside your child, cradling her close the way it warms your heart and sweetens motherhood to do. Around the bed, a line of children coils, watching and waiting to sleep beside the babe. Each gives you fifty sticky palm-warm cents to pay for the privilege that should be yours alone, to nestle the tiny body soft and damp and limp with sleep.

The baby cries. You wake and rise to feed her. After she is settled in your arms and sucking, you raise the blind a cautious inch or two to watch how morning whitens the bay, the mountain and the dunes, a thousand childish pines calligraphed black on the rice paper sky. You stroke the baby's downy head. Sleep, love.

The young man wants you. It is no mockery. You are worth wanting, young yourself, and slim, hair flowing to your waist, your breasts an ornament, belly flat and pale and luminous as morning on the river. Your hands are young, your throat young, eyes clear, thighs firm, wrists young, knees young, ears young, ankles and toes and waist young, lust young. You have a mother and are not a mother. The young man's touch is radiant over your buttocks, across the curved space of your back.

The baby cries. You wake and rise to feed her. Across the room, the man in the bed artlessly unfurls his naked limbs, sighs, ascending toward daytime, anticipating the summons of the clock that will make him disappear. Covers kicked away, you see his chest, where you want to rest your head, the arms, sleep-sprawled, you want to feel around you, and will the baby to eat fast so you can go to him and be with him a moment, only that, before he leaves.

The clock goes off. The man obeys it, emptying your bed, and there is no time for mothering of mothers, for the touching of fathers.

You rock in your chair beside the window and feed the child until she sleeps.

LAURA CHESTER

from: *Primagravida* _____

By the third day of recovery, dusk time, the baby lies suckling as I lie on my side. Room lights off, only the country air, the open window and the dim light of spring, first buds and first breeze and first swallow full branches over by the local highschool, swooping their song, their night come alive calls, and the purple hyacinth by my elbow comes and goes in its quiet luxurious perfume as the curtains blow and I know I've reached some other shore. That Geoff reached it with me. That I'm lying here now with part of my own body, part of us, but so apart, connected for a lifetime, after the life line, after the breast is gone and divisions are made, I'll hold this evening like a quiver, knowing that the body doesn't always give so easily, that it must lose what it holds, alluvial, come floating back from the sharpest distance, washed up on the opening fan. Baby's drinking so fast, he has to stop to catch his breath. Then back to the nipple and his sigh-song. This first. This brand new spring. Clovis curls in.

oo oo oo

DAPHNE MARLATT

from: Rings, v. _____

Hungry? Yes, it's time.
                       & light. Wind's blowing
the curtain, see, patterns of light like waves falling
across the floor. & cool now on my skin, unbuttoning
blouse, evaporates, my sweat from the sun gone. You?
cold? The cotton blanket, all your things, that delicate
smell you're wrapt in, new. But you must smell the
grass on me, sweat, insects, earth? These things you'll
spend hours with. All right, i'm hurrying. & the milk's
already dripping. That's your world. Hunger surge, mouth
open already crying. pain? There, into the rocking chair's
familiar fabric against my back, elbow up to support your
head, & nipple lifted towards. You're drinking now, those
hungry sucking movements of mouth, palate like little fish.
And snuggling down myself into the chairback can relax now,
So, The day is still,
            Again,
                  This world. Something precious,
something out of the course of time marked off by clocks.
Wind blows, plants breathe out their odours drawn by sun,
drifts, gradually over the house, shadows the back lane
lengthen, birds too, active at different times remark,
their wings worm's activity, the day's age ... daze, an
age was all i knew, child in blue sea dress & bare legs,
climbing from terrace to terrace. Uncalled (from home),
called, by the focus of an orchid, length of tree shadow,
sun a glint on sea below, the island light, passing from
mainland out, to sea, to see *where* time turns, known by
intensity of odours, orchids', & the earth here,

                            Here's
lilacs outside your window. Lilac time i brought you home in.
Thick fragrance up the back lane our car drove thru, Al
drove thru, ecstacy, to be outdoors again, get out on grass,
springy, unlike cement or hospital floors my feet had known
a week, & you had never known it, smelt, the sun. in every
blade, leaf, culm. breathing light. & never known the

lilacs i'd thought old lady flowers a dying, virulent as
fever (ecstasy

      Cold at my heart (*must co-o-me down*),
times you're so quiet (sleeping) when i bend can't tell if
you're breathing still. & Al: of course he is. The cats,
Conch in your crib the other day. by suffocation. sudden
death. Wake up suddenly past the hour you should have woken
cried for milk, Come running down the hall, fear at my throat,
The time, the time it takes to reach your door, open it,
draw near (slow motion, slow, reluctant) Find you sleeping
still.
   The fear.
        Stops. Up my heart, stops breath. Stop
the circle (*spinning thru, Drop, all you troubles by the
river, side, Catch a painted pony on the spinning wheel ride.*)
Which does spring on thru. It's fear of the unexpected, of
the music suddenly broken off. It's fear of it happening
When . . . ? ('Is the music over, Mom?')

    Let the spinning wheel spin.

                & the pressure
built up til it hurts in the other breast, is full, towel
tucked under wet, & you, long hard pulls now, almost empty,
time to shift you. Lift you up, little head on my shoulder,
stroke that burp that never comes between times, only after,
only they say, burp him between breasts, & i grow tired of
hurting, & you, maybe want some more, or maybe fall asleep,
already? I put you down in my arm, left side i never can
arrange it right, so your nose is free to breathe & your
head not turned in some way awkward as the other never is.
Left side, sinistra. But you're eager. No need to suck,
it's there, drip from the nipple, tho you do, must, i figure,
your gulping that swift, spurt, like a water fountain down
your throat.
      Connect. Open conduit, light or liquid flowing
thru. you. in the circle my arms make around you drinking
sun, my own, skin, hair absorbed, what you now take in. all
that you need.
      Tho it seemed so thin-looking when it first
came, in a milky water. all the nutrients are there. &

still it runs. more as you want more, grow more. Amazed,
at the interconnection still. Those first days how, with
every suck, i could feel the walls of uterus contract. You,
isolate now, & born, healing my body for me.

oo oo oo

FRANCES JAFFER

from: Milk Song _____

venus venom the long loss

is it the great beauty she hears the lullaby
the wide song the lap

the lost sweet curve of milk the
rubber squeak the melody drains

into dark she throws it back the mouthful
the mistake

the dying the almost dead

through the last tiny finger the milky
the tiny living

milky song

healer voice
rocking

lying in milk the baby the sick

venom *she could not atone*
striking the great gone blue-red

Mother

to strive for to win to strive

to lose

. . .

Bye-Lo Baby Mommy's gone

to wrap you

upside down in the head
of the hearth-warming woolly

sheep dancing over
nightly stiles into a

sump

        the blue cow stands
        in the way and the sheep

        go freely over the field

. . .

waves rise for the moon milky

curling singing this moment is day
and will be until night:

healer
voice rocking

        when the earth unbends it won't go
        without me

JANE LAZARRE

from: *The Mother Knot* _____

I felt I should never have had a baby. If anyone had told me what it would be like, I might have saved my life in time. Who was this immensely powerful person, screaming unintelligibly, sucking my breast until I was in a state of fatigue the likes of which I had never known? Who was he and by what authority had he claimed the right to my life? I would never be a good mother. Hadn't I already caused him to be colicky with my own treacherous anxiety? The experts were right, I thought. Babies are born to be placid, contented creatures. It is only the bad mother repressing her unfair resentment, holding the baby too tightly, too loosely, too often, too rarely, letting him cry, picking him up too soon, feeding him too much, too little, suffocating him with her love or not loving him enough—it is only the bad mother who is to blame.

How, I wondered, had I ever blamed my parents for anything?

I hugged my sweater tightly around me. No belly to get in the way. Though I was still ten pounds heavier than my usual weight, I felt positively gaunt. I was so thankful not to be pregnant any more, I laughed and stroked my body which now belonged only to me once again. I might diet without worrying about fetal nutrition; I might exercise until I dropped—only I would be fatigued. Then I felt my blouse dampen with the sweet, clear milk. It was time for Benjamin to eat. I ran all the way home waiting impatiently for the feel of his smooth little cheek against my breast.

His mouth, vulnerable and innocent at other times, grabbed my nipple and sucked it into himself with a ferocity, a knowledgeability, which was awesome in its purity. I had never before been in contact with such driven instinct. After only several days of his life, we both felt that the breast was his. As he drew the milk out of me, my inner self seemed to shrink into a very small knot, gathering intensity under a protective shell, moving away, further and further away, from the changes being wrought by this child who was at once separate and a part of me. Frightened that he would claim my life completely, I desperately tried to cling to my boundaries. Yet I held him very close, stroked his skin, imagined that we were still one person.

I turned to that self inside of me, that girlwoman who had once been all I needed to know of myself, whom I had fought to understand, to love, to free—I turned to her now and I banished her. Into a protective shell tied in a knot, she retreated, four, five, six times a day, whenever Benjamin wanted to nurse. Soon, even when I sought her, she would not come, but began to stay out of reach longer and longer, sometimes not reappearing for whole days. For if she was present when the baby needed me, she was of necessity pushed aside, sent to go hungry. She who had been my life, whom I knew I had to nourish daily in order to be fed in return, hid for weeks, hoarding her gentleness and her strength, placing no gifts in my outstretched hands.

In my arms, I held my baby. After he drank from me, sometimes he would sleep. I stayed still for hours then, staring at his face, comparing his toes to mine, finding a turn of his mouth which reminded me of my sister's, discovering in the shape of his torso the suggestion of his father's body. Every detail of his face seemed, like a photograph taken many years before, to ring with the tones of my own features. I was always looking for something familiar, a prospector searching for a treasure which would set the world right.

At other times, during and after feedings, he would cry and scream. I would walk him through the house, weeping with him for my incompetence, apologizing for my anxious and jittery soul, which was clearly the wrong style for good mothers. Sometimes I hated him for rejecting me so completely; "Shut up! I'll kill myself if you don't shut up!" I'd yell. Then I would try to shove my nipple into his mouth and he would push it away, his face distorted with pain.

I'd put him in the carriage so as not to harm him with my tentacles of rage, and I'd sit huddled on the couch, door slammed unsuccessfully against his cries, holding my ears and moaning with loss. And in the corner of my desk, my typewriter and my record books sat silently, mocking me through layers of dust.

When he had cried long enough to subdue my anger, I held him and rocked him again until he became quiet. I checked his breathing, kissed his lips, his eyes, warding off the spirit of psychosis and, mercifully, he was willing to suck. I held him close as our dark eyes met, telling him silently, Suck, darling, take me, use me to grow. Live, My Life, and love me, love me, while I try desperately to love you.

oo oo oo

ALICIA OSTRIKER

Letter to M. _____

Dear M. I am writing to thank you for the gift of the pipe, and your kind note, "Lactation with representation," which has given me some midnight chuckles. I have, you will be interested to know—as a mother of three and a graduate student of English literature—been redeeming the time I spend with Gabriel in the rocking chair. He is the sweetest thing, intense at first, then dribbling and snoozing, but of course they all were. Possibly because he is my last, and when this phase is finished I will be that much closer to the stupor and the letting go, I am thinking about the erotic pleasure of nursing.

You remember, I hope. To see them visibly grow, fed by us—it is almost too much. And then the sensation itself, like a cat lapping; only we are the innocent cat. You remember?

I don't believe I have ever seen a discussion of this experience; or indeed, any mention of the idea that we can be sexually aroused by being suckled, and that suckling is (biologically must be, just as orgasm during intercourse for a man must be, to insure survival of the species) physically pleasurable, one of the most pleasurable things it is possible for a human to do. Why do we not say this? Why are mothers always represented sentimentally, as having some sort of altruistically self-sacrificing "maternal" feelings, as if they did not enjoy themselves? Is it so horrible if we enjoy ourselves; another love that dare not tell its name?

oo oo oo

ALICIA OSTRIKER

The Cambridge Afternoon was Grey _____

When you were born, the nurse's aide
Wore a grey uniform, and in general
The place was starched

To a kind of religious ecstasy.
They brought you, struggling feebly
Inside the cotton blanket, only your eyes

Were looking as if you already knew
What thought and love were going to be like
And this of course was making your eyes brim

With laughter, like some child
Who's been hiding in a closet
Among the woolen overcoats while the anxious parents

Call *Where are you?* At the right moment the child
Bounces into the room
Pretending innocence ... My hot breast

Was delighted, and ran up to you like a dog
To a younger dog it wants to make friends with
So the scandalized aide had to pull the grey

Curtains around our bed, making a sound
Of hissing virtue, curtainrings on rod,
While your eyes were saying *Where am I? I'm here!*

oo oo oo

CAROLE ITTER

Cry Baby _____

It is visiting hours. Four new mothers receive scores of visitors. Each mother has put on her make-up ahead of time and arranged herself into the most comfortable seated position possible considering the stitches. Some of the mothers make more than one trip to the nursery with groups of visitors to look at the new arrival. When my second group of visitors arrive, I decide also to show this new baby to them. I shuffle down the hallway and for the first time look through the glass window. I can't tell which baby is mine and they are all crying and I can't stand it so I go back to the room and crawl into bed. The next day I try it alone. I stand on one side of the glass, crying, and the baby is on the other side of the glass, crying, and we are not able to get together because it is not 'time'. I recall Oscar, the farmer saying that after the calf is born, many farmers remove the calf from the cow for the first two days. It provides the distance between them that the cow needs in order to stop worrying about her offspring. Is that the role hospitals offer to new mothers? I leave with the baby on the second day.

Sputters, growls, bubbles, bigger than any journal-keeping reality. Time measured by the emptiness of a tummy to the fullness of these breasts, then reversed. I have never known tiredness like this, as though travelling day coach from Vancouver to Halifax to Vancouver to Halifax to Vancouver, two weeks of it, two weeks old today, not more than three continuous hours of sleep, my dreams rich, strange: he brings newborn kittens one by one into the bed, wet, crawling over my skin while the mother cat is crying out, I call his name but only the first letter comes, *Gee*, screaming and awake.

Sleeps, sucks, shits and belches, is very strong and has the paternal dimple on a pointed chin, the eyes are steady, this is our child. *Hi there. I'm your mom. That guy? He's your dad. Your name? Well, we like the sound of it, hope it works for you. We weren't very good at finding you a name, long list, old relatives, ancestors. We'll find another name for you too, one less feminine, more sturdy, the kind you can use should you become an economist or a revolutionist or a writer. Like Welwyn. Or Marden. I'm your mom and I'm full of magic tricks and milk.*

He and I celebrate an anniversary by taking a short walk together, arriving back just a little bit early. The baby is quiet, upstairs listening to grandmother coo and soothe. We have some extra time, I carry the jar of vaseline, he the rubber prophylactic towards the bed. I am talking nervously, what if it doesn't work, isn't possible? and, it isn't. I begin talking more nervously, he long and straight, says sharply, *don't talk about it.* Better I get up, baby is hungry and needing a bath, crud and fluff stuck in the armpits, the neck, an empty belly. (*Later,* says grandmother, *you'll wonder how you ever did it.*) Well, the month was a miserable failure with this beautiful wee child responding to the tension in me, the total exhaustion, the colic night after night, the screeching for hours on end.

"Colic is a bad break to get with a first baby; it
shatters so much of the natural joy new parents share."

The exhaustion. The depression, the tension, the visitors, the telephone, the hemorrhoids, the stitches, the dreams, the stomach flu, the sleeplessness. The colic, the grip water, the barley water, the bottled water, the pacifier, hot water bottle, and then the tranquillizers casually prescribed for what? *A three week old baby?* exclaimed the pharmacist, the father, the grandmother, the aunt. NO WAY. The laundries, the typesetting home business, the clients, the Christmas, the family with three children who had stomach flu and staph infection who moved in for the Christmas season. Quite literally, the longest months I've known, the hours awake.

". . . and if your baby's crying half the night, making evenings
with your husband hideous, destroying everyone's sleep, you'll
be ready to try anything that might stop it. Sometimes warming, cuddling, rocking, or (strictly by prescription) sedatives or
a change of formula will do it. It's not temper, it's pain."

Baby child, holding me on the line. Tension, then no milk or restless milk, breasts that are needed, the connection so distant as I look down at the bare head, the embryonic profile so exquisitely contoured, one brilliant eye open which looks up at me. The nipple held fully in the small mouth, the tongue sucking rhythmically five or six times then a brief rest, then twanging the tip of the nipple quickly and on again.

When I leave the house, I forget that other very insistent existence. Yet two hours away and I'm feeling my breasts fill up suddenly and I'm fretting. Can this presence be part of the next, what, fifteen years of my life, this insistence. I don't think I'll be able to do it, I simply won't be able to cope.

Growls, farts, grunts, groans, squeals, every few seconds another loop of sound, the audio version of what's happening inside. The baby lies in the adjacent room in the old wicker carriage, the noises are atrocious. I should be asleep. The public health nurse said most firmly, *When the baby sleeps, you sleep.* But baby is restless as I am. My thoughts to my stomach, and then to my breasts, then to that stomach, then the sound of that crying, stomach, breast, stomach, a constant refilling.

One of his friends phones, then phones back to ask of the baby. *Grand.* Asks if I breastfeed. *Yes.* Asks how do I like it? *Weird.* Well, it was a weird question to begin with. How to expound further by telephone, that she lies at my breast sucking? That my milk gives her colic and therefore pain? That she screams for hours on end? That I don't love her then? That I'm at my wits end and nobody has noticed? I pick up a book I've been trying to read, stand in the partial afternoon light while pushing the carriage back and forth with the other hand. That way the cries don't hurt.

> "Colic is defined as a 'paroxysm of acute abdominal pain,' but we are not sure just what it is other than a separate and distinct pattern which is commonly referred to as 'colic' or 'the three months' colic. (If it lasted more than three months, we would find lots of mothers in the funny farm.)"

He said, *Doesn't it ever make you angry?* Baby was squealing and screeching and squirming on my lap. *How can it, she's doing this because she's uncomfortable.*

The crying is almost continuous from 7:30 at night to 7:30 in the morning. My stomach aches and cramps, I hold back screaming out, doubled over in the pain. If that tummy cramps as mine does, no wonder the crying. I am exhausted and angry at everyone. I am too tired to sleep, too weak to eat and there's no food in the house. I make an appointment to see the doctor and as I enter the office, he looks at me and smiles, giving his immediate diagnosis—*It's the case of the exhausted mother and the thriving baby.* He prescribes librium and says that once my sleep gets back in order, so should everything else. I am breast feeding and probably shouldn't be taking drugs, it might affect the milk. Perhaps this is a blessing in disguise. Within a week, I am totally dependent on the librium for a night's sleep and guard the tablets carefully. My sanity is being rescued and I am so grateful that they work. A month later I can see that there is a baby and I am a mother and we are inseparable and I love this babe beyond description.

Laughs, smiles at everybody and every thing, knows the family, reaches out for things, knows three toys, cried when he left the room, is amazed, simply amazed by the family cat. A little person, distinct as the two ears which stick out so far they sometimes fold over. The longest three months of my life. My feelings so mixed, loving the baby yet despising the time consumed. I now can find one hour a day to spend at the home business. I am still tired all the time, no strength, no stamina.

> "Postpartum depression is now considered to be the reaction of a vulnerable personality to the stresses and strains of pregnancy and delivery, followed by the responsibility to a new baby ... the sufferer feels continually tired with a persistent headache, and aches and pains all over her body. She becomes increasingly prone to feelings of inadequacy ..."

The crying doesn't stop and I've got to do something that is a diversion from the sound. The book says that you let the baby cry itself to sleep at night, you do not go to it and that the first night you try this, the baby will cry for an hour, then the second night, for a half hour, the third night for fifteen minutes and then not at all. I will follow the book as nothing else is working and the first night, this baby cries for an hour, the second night the baby cries for two hours, the third night the baby cries for three hours and the fourth night, the baby cries for four hours. The book does not work. I am in some kind of deep agony, I listen to the advice of everyone, I don't know what to do. The most sensible advice from a neighbour, that a baby will fall asleep once it is content. This one isn't. Others talk of spoiled babies, how they will cry because they know they'll get picked up. I understand the resentment that parents feel when a baby cries all the time and also the guilt. I can't stand the crying. Every night the crying. Is it fear of the long sleep? Is it hunger? She is hungry but won't eat, is tired but won't sleep. Then somehow, finally, whew, the crying has stopped, I take a deep breath in the silence. A phone call had interrupted the emptying of the right breast, a client for the home typesetting business arrived during the left one. Each evening comes and I am tired and tired of being continuously tired. I don't have the option to sleep.

Silence is the absence of a crying baby. Maybe I'm going out of my mind, deeper and deeper into depression. I am too isolated or I am lonely or, I want a whole afternoon to myself or, I want to see more people or nobody drops in, so I work all day yet don't take time for myself. I've lost contact with him, we live on different shifts. I see that he does what he wants to do when he feels like doing it and that I do what's needed to be done. If this is where marriage begins to break down, then I know it. Three days went by when he didn't touch the baby.

> "Not surprisingly, the first few weeks at home can be the most difficult time of a mother's life. . . . However good your intentions to put child, husband and home first, as a new mother you are courting trouble if you forget that you too, have needs . . ."

It's the disillusion. Each day there is less of me and more of the baby. I don't read anything, books or newspapers. Mostly I am exhausted creatively and that's the largest problem; being strongly motivated in a direction other than motherhood yet finding motherhood is totally consuming with no releases. To collect whatever is myself at the end of the day is about as interesting or possible as collecting raindrops from the windowpane.

I begin to think that having a baby is some sort of trick played on me. I am grounded, immobilized, everything halts while this baby takes what it needs to grow. I resent all those voices ringing in my ears, *Oh, you* should *have a baby, you'd make a great mother*. Now I think they were wrong, that motherhood is a difficult role, that I've made a dreadful mistake. (Years later, she, so bright-eyed, is to say, *Oh, you're the best mother in the whole world* and I reply *Thanks, kid* thinking what can she remember of what we went through.) I didn't have a baby in order to have a baby, I had a baby in order to have a child.

BABIES, WHO COULD HURT THEM

He told me the story of that phrase scrawled in black paint on the wall behind the crib and I know how that mother felt. Firstly, babies like fat people best and since I'm not fat and cuddly to lay on, they tend to fuss more quickly, all those bones sticking out, not enough soft parts, where's the tits for milk?

HERE IT IS, MOMMY'S TIT, DON'T CRY BABY, WE'LL GET IT IN YOUR MOUTH AND THEN EVERYTHING WILL BE ALL RIGHT. OH BABY, STOP IT. STOP IT. OH BABY, WAIT A MINUTE, THE NURSING PAD IS CAUGHT IN THE NURSING BRA. OH POOR BABY HAS TO WAIT WHILE MOMMY FIGURES THIS OUT, DON'T CRY LITTLE BABY, SOON IT WILL BE ALL BETTER AND YOU WILL HAVE SOME MILK FOR YOUR

TUMMY AND A TIT FOR YOUR MOUTH, THERE—IT'S FREE. HERE'S WHAT YOU'VE BEEN WAITING FOR, BABY, WHAT A GOOD BABY.

OH, BABY IS HUNGRY, BABY DOESN'T WANT TO GO TO SLEEP YET. BABY WANTS TO SUCK SOME MORE. HOW COULD BABY STILL BE HUNGRY? BUT BABY IS CRYING SO IT MUST BE HUNGRY. WE WILL SIT DOWN AGAIN SO THAT BABY CAN SUCK. THERE.

BABY'S HUNGRY AGAIN. BABY WAS SUCKING THE MILK FROM THE TIT JUST HALF AN HOUR AGO BUT BABY'S HUNGRY AGAIN. BABY IS SUCKING THE MILK EVERY TWO HOURS AND SOMETIMES EVEN MORE FREQUENTLY BUT BABY MUST GAIN WEIGHT THEREFORE BABY MUST SUCK THE MILK WHENEVER BABY FRETS. BABY DOESN'T CRY BECAUSE NOBODY CAN STAND TO LISTEN TO BABY CRY, ESPECIALLY BABY'S MOMMY. EVEN BEFORE BABY CRIES, MOMMY GIVES BABY THE TIT. BUT THE TIT MUST BE WASHED FIRST AND BABY'S SHAT ITS DIAPER SO THAT HAS TO BE CHANGED AS WELL BECAUSE BABY MIGHT GET COLD SITTING IN ITS SHIT, SO BABY WILL BE CHANGED JUST AS SOON AS MOMMY WASHES HER TITS AND *THEN* BABY CAN SUCK THE MILK FROM THE TIT. BABY HAS NO IDEA HOW CLEAN IT IS, WILL BABY EVER KNOW HOW CLEAN IT IS, WILL BABY CARE?

The best thing about being a baby is that it doesn't last too long, only a short period of immobility, total dependency, poor articulation and poof! it's over, and a more tangible reality can be faced. I don't for one moment imagine that those who project a sort of Buddhist serenity and all-encompassing understanding onto a young baby are those who are also getting up two or three times a night to tend its needs or hanging over a wringer washer.

So much changes as the baby grows. Crying now and I don't agonize while it happens nor resent my days. Crawls for long periods each day, plays with toys and other simple objects, occasionally looking at me to see what I am doing. The exhaustion is leaving slowly and with it, the depression. The baby is still crying, maybe I can help. The crying is part of the baby; apart from the baby, the crying parts the baby, it's partly the crying.

Anyone who has been a mother can hear any child crying sooner than anyone else, have you noticed? I hear a young baby next door. The baby has been crying hysterically. There are moments of exhausted sobbings and then continuously piercing wails. I doubt the baby is being tortured but that's how it sounds. It rarely cries for so long. My feelings go out to the family who are in such close range to the screeching. Suddenly it is silent and minutes later, a brief choking sound. Silence as the absence of a baby crying.

In the mornings, I remember to take a vitamin B and some iron tablets, right after the porridge. Baby plays on the floor, bumping against the chair, then knocking the chair to get the feel of it. Mornings are slow, in fact awful and it's not really very early. Baby sleeps longest between 5 am and 9 am, comes into bed for the breast and then we play until her father can't take anymore of it, having gone to bed only a few hours earlier. Sometimes in his sleep, he mutters *go away, go away*. Other times he says *fuck off, why dontcha?*, but he's usually quite pleasant about it. Mornings are slow. The baby bumps the chair again and cries while trying to pull up. She'll be walking soon enough. I change the wet diaper, find some woolen pants, put on the socks and slippers, tuck in the shirt meanwhile baby hollers and kicks and tries to get away, all the while firmly pinned to the floor by my knee.

The porridge got made and served. Baby won't eat it. I take baby out of the chair, wipe hands and face, clean off the plastic bib, hang it to dry, collect the uneaten cold porridge from the tray and put it in the fridge, wipe down the chair, put it away, fold up the newspapers from under it and throw them away, wipe off the floor where the porridge was tossed just further than the newspapers. Breakfast is over. I sit down and hope there will be ten whole minutes before I have to move again. Each day the needs are immediate and basic and terribly repetitive.

Much of it blotted out, wiped off, slated clean. The baby cried and cried and cried and I said firmly and resolutely never never never again will I go through these months. Baby cried and cried and cried. Baby would sleep for an hour, cry for two hours and suck for one hour, then sleep for an hour, cry for two and suck for one. One night I stepped from the bed and collapsed to the floor, a couple of thunks against the wall and down.

One night this is what happened. I was standing by the kitchen sink, having already laid out in front of me a clean tea towel, some paper serviettes and a sharp paring knife on top of the neatly folded pile. I wasn't awake. What woke me up was him walking up and saying wryly, *What are you going to do, peel the baby?* That's when I woke up. I looked at what I'd laid out in front of me in amazement and quickly put the items away and went to the crying baby. It's taken time pondering just what I was about to do and what might have happened had he not walked in the door at that point. I did not know what I was doing. I did not know what I was doing.

Everything seems different this morning. Something is about to happen, something startling or maybe just exciting. A change in the air, in my mind, something I woke up with and have carried since. Here I am, living about a mile and a half from the hospital in which I was born, anything could be a change. What is it that hangs in my mind like a trick toy? The baby yells for the milk which sits in a cup on the counter, the demand-shout "yu" means milk. Out of the chair and she begins to crawl back to eat the lumps of porridge that she methodically dropped onto the floor. Now I remember. The biggest thing that will happen today is that the telephone service man will arrive to install another extension onto the phone. That makes three phone lines and two extensions, five phones in this rambling house in the far end of town. If we can't be near our friends, at least we are near our telephones. Baby is learning to pull up against the chair. Baby needs my conversation, my voice talking and I am unable to keep up the patter, baby simply wishing to be recognized and I know that, but how much talking do I have to do?

Wow, are you ever lovely. What a lovely baby you are. Just look at you looking at the tit. Hey there, beauty, got a smile? Ssssmmmmiiiiile? Oh now, that's it, thatsa smile. What a good lookin' kid you are. Hey there, got another smile for mommy?

MADELINE TIGER

"Men also look in mirrors, experience troublesome and delicious sensations, contribute to the generation of species, and ride throughout their lifetimes the tide of emotions influenced by glandular secretions . . . precisely as rooted in nature as women . . . Will women begin comparing the bodies of men to flowers?"
—*Alicia Ostriker*, Stealing the Language

For My Sons Who Had Mouths Like Rosebuds ___

who begged me years later not to cut the oak down
for that had been the shade of the room of night milk
and such soft noises, and I had to cut the oak down
so I stare at the air where the huge heavy tree rose
straight up out of weed among azaleas and into the height
high above our house, right before our eyes,
with nothing else in view but sky and lamplight
and the blackbird,   the suddenly overgrown oak tree
and you

who squawled imperiously out of sleep
out of the deep sweat
exhaustions pulling me past the ropes of my own
vulnerable rug-raft and temporary pillows

whose fists made sugary
grooves on my flesh like
the steps of little bears
across moonscapes

your noses fat pulps, reddening, you
all full of waiting, breathless and
tense while I changed your soaked diapers
and swaddled you tightly

little pigs come little pigs
drums of hunger
stretches of wind in
stretches of sweet fat
taut over drum ribs
and plump arms and plump legs

and plump bottoms and tribal
drum-bellies and all waiting
on the edge
of howl
on the edge
of sharp
crying
on the edge of nerve and need
and the mouths
groping for my
nipple while
I helped you find
me find me find
this   source

at my sources, milk and the whole spirit
whatever I was whatever I was with-
holding, your mouths made such quick work
with me and then your eyes were shining
up into my bent face, your eyes
just before sleep so open then shining
they gave me back Yes, the night
sky glass pools, Lac St. Pierre blue
to the bottom,   there   there   thus with
the sucking glazed into the
absolute absence of anything but.

Then we became content; so love is
born, that is just how it is born,
love is born out of utter
hunger, then the mouth
becoming muscular to
take and take as much
milk as desire requires,
drawing all the world of nourishment while
the eyes tell back luminous volumes and then close
and the mouth softens again again it is a rose

oo oo oo

JOAN SLESINGER LOGGHE

Empty Breasts _____

I want to take a walk about empty breasts.
Unless you have had full ones
you cannot fathom.
My baby girl at two
knows the taste of empty breasts.
All weekend you came onto me,
the seeds shattered,
all at once it smelled
like empty breasts.

Only once in life
is a last child weaned
at age forty
on the notes of a flute
sounding empty.
All over Wisconsin, farmers
are smiling like yogurt,
gone broke, gone sour
by the river, Empty Breasts.
They rub the udders of Holsteins
with Bag Balm from its green can
with red flowers. The heifers
breathe an interlude
of empty clover breath.

All night I called you.
And did you come?
Nothing arrived except myself
wearing a purple sweater
over my newly empty breasts.
Full full girl of Pittsburgh,
enticing college girl of Chicago,
Boston girls growing libraries for teeth,
nothing prepared you for this.

I want to engorge like a mother
gone suddenly ebony statue
in the Folk Art museums of Africa.

I want to tell all the women of America
to mourn for these empty breasts.
To speak like a whisper of linen.
To dance like the wagging finger
beckoning me toward change of life.

Crossing America in covered wagons,
the train centered around itself.
Women swap stories, flip flapjacks.
Men's laughter comes in from the dark
like buffalo. It is time to break camp,
pick up the reins,
move on out.

FURTHER MOTHERING

oo oo oo

RACHEL HADAS

Two and One ─────────────────────

Asleep between us
(father, mother
pushing a stroller)
this treasure is.

Gain from loss.
Good-bye, speech;
here in reach
is Paradise

(here in the park,
the dogs, the dirt,
my milky shirt,
cries in the dark)—

was all along?
Yes and no.
Until I had you
I had it wrong.

The focus given—
an infant's face—
they are one place,
Hell and Heaven.

We lose to find.
Youth, beauty,
wave good-bye.
I bend my mind,

strike my temple,
try to grapple
with the riddle,
yet it's simple:

Janus-face,
here you are.
You light up space
like a single star.

On either side
an emptiness—
here Born, there Died—
fills the place

yet fades away
in the glow
of a single day.
I know, I know:

You weren't always here.
And you'll go. (When?)
You'll disappear.
Birth/death: twin

mirrors reflecting
only each other
over the sleeping
head in the stroller

lose their power,
pale in one
brilliant hour
of living sun.

Brush of a wing—
or is it blade?—
flickering
over what we've made,

that angel love,
enormous knife,
wing of a dove
scoring life

swoops its shadow
invisibly
into a meadow
where we three,

mother, father,
baby, lie
close together
under the sky.

Trees are in flower.
Grass is green.
The hour is noon
and is forever.

LYDIA DAVIS

from: What You Learn _____

Idle

You learn how to be idle, how to do nothing. That is the new thing in your life—to do nothing. To do nothing and not be impatient about doing nothing. It is easy to do nothing and become impatient. It is not easy to do nothing and not mind it, not mind the hours passing, the hours of the morning passing and then the hours of the afternoon, and one day passing and the next passing, while you do nothing.

What You Can Count On

You learn never to count on anything being the same from day to day, that he will fall asleep at a certain hour, or sleep for a certain length of time. Some days he sleeps for several hours at a stretch, other days he sleeps no more than half an hour.

Sometimes he will wake suddenly crying hard, when you were prepared to go on working another hour. Now you prepare to stop. But as it takes you a few minutes to end your work for the day, and you cannot go to him immediately, he stops crying and continues quiet. Now, though you have prepared to end work for the day, you resume working.

Sitting Still

You learn to be patient. You learn to stare as he stares, to stare up at the rafters as long as he stares up at the rafters, sitting still in a large space.

Renunciation

You give up, or postpone, for his sake, many of the pleasures you once enjoyed, such as eating meals when you are hungry, eating as much as you want, watching a movie all the way through from beginning to end, reading as much of a book as you want to at one sitting, going to sleep when you are tired, sleeping until you have had enough sleep.

At a party you have been looking forward to as you never used to look forward to a party, now that you are at home alone with him so much, you will not be able to talk to anyone for more than a few minutes, because he cries so constantly, and in the end he will be your only company, in a back bedroom.

Odd Things You Notice about Him

The dark gray lint that collects in the lines of his palm.

The white fuzz that collects in his armpit.

The black under the tips of his fingernails: you have let his nails get too long, because it is hard to make a precise cut on such a small thing constantly moving. Now it would take a very small nailbrush to clean them.

When he yawns, how the wings of his nose turn yellow.

When he holds his breath and pushes down on his diaphragm, how quickly his face turns red.

His uneven breath: how his breath changes in response to his motion, to his curiosity.

How his bent arms and legs, when he is asleep on his stomach, take the shape of an hourglass.

When he lies against your chest, how he lifts his head to look around like a turtle and drops it again because it is so heavy.

The colors of his face: his pink forehead, his bluish eyelids, his reddish-gold eyebrows. And the tiny beads of sweat standing out from the tiny pores of his skin.

How his hands move slowly through the air like crabs or other sea creatures before closing on a toy.

Connected by a Single Nipple

You are lying on the bed nursing him but you are not holding onto him with your arms or hands and he is not holding onto you. He is connected to you by a single nipple.

Disorder

You learn that there is less order in your life now. Or if there is to be order, you must work harder at maintaining it than you once did, or you will find yourself in a situation of disorder. For instance, it is evening and you are lying on the bed with the baby half asleep beside you watching *Casablanca*. Suddenly a thunderstorm breaks and the rain comes down hard. You remember the baby's clothes out on the line, and you get up from the bed and run outdoors. The baby begins crying at being left so abruptly half asleep on the bed. *Casablanca* continues, the baby screams now, and you are out in the hard rainfall in your white bathrobe taking many small clothes off the line.

Distraction

You decide you must attend some public event, say a concert, despite the difficulty of arranging such a thing. You make elaborate preparations to leave the baby with a babysitter, taking a bag full of equipment, a folding bed, a folding stroller, and so on. Now, as the concert proceeds, you sit thinking not about the concert, but only about the elaborate preparations you made and whether they have been adequate, and no matter how often you try to listen to the concert, you will hear only a few minutes of it before thinking again about those elaborate preparations and whether they have been adequate to the comfort of the baby and the convenience of the babysitter.

You Do Not Know When He Will Fall Asleep

If his eyes are wide open staring at a light, it does not mean he will not be asleep within minutes.

If he cries with a squeaky cry and squirms with wiry strength against your chest, digging his sharp little fingernails into your shoulder, or raking your neck, or pushing his face into your shirt, it does not mean he will not relax in five minutes and grow heavy. But five minutes is a very long time when you are caring for a baby.

Why He Smiles

He looks at a window with serious interest. He looks at a painting and smiles. It is hard to know what that smile means. Is he pleased by the painting? Is the painting funny to him? No, soon you understand that he smiles at the painting for the same reason he smiles at you: because the painting is looking at him.

A Problem of Balance

A problem of balance: if he yawns, he falls over backwards.

Time

It is not that five minutes is always a very long time when you are caring for a baby but that time passes very slowly when you are waiting for a baby to go to sleep, when you are listening to him cry alone in his bed or whimper close to your ear.

Then time passes very briskly once the baby is asleep. You have your breakfast, and twenty minutes is gone, you shower and another twenty minutes is gone, you wash some dishes and pick up some things in the living room and another twenty minutes is gone, and now, just as you are ready to think of doing some work, the baby is awake again.

The things you have to do have always taken this long to do, but before the baby was born it did not matter, because there were many such hours in the day to do such things. Now there is only one hour, and again later, on some days, one hour, and again, very late in the day, on some days, one last hour.

Moving Forward

You worry about moving forward, or about the difference between moving forward and staying in one place. You begin to notice which things have to be done over and over again in one day, and which things have to be done once every day, and which things have to be done every few days, and which every week, and which every month, and which every six months, and all these things have to do with marking time, staying in one place, rather than moving forward, or rather making sure things do not slip backward, whereas certain other things are done only once. A job to earn money is done only once, a letter is written saying a thing only once and never again, an event is planned that will happen only once, news is received or news passed along only once, and if, in this way, something happens that will happen only once, this day is different from other days, and on this day your life seems to move forward, and it is easier to sit still holding the baby and staring at the wall knowing that on this day, at least, your life has moved forward, there has been a change, however small.

Patience

You try to understand why on some days you have no patience and on others your patience is limitless and you will stand over him for a long time where he lies on the changing table on his back waving his arms, kicking his legs, or looking up at a painting on the wall and smiling. Why on some days it is limitless and on others, or at other times, late in a day when you have been patient, you cannot bear his crying and want to threaten to put him away in his bed to cry alone if he does not stop crying in your arms, and sometimes you do put him away in his bed to cry alone.

Paradox

You begin to understand paradox: lying on the bed next to him, you are deeply interested, watching his face and holding his hands, and yet at the same time you are deeply bored, wishing you were somewhere else doing something else: it is as though the interest lay at the heart of the boredom or the boredom lay at the heart of the interest.

Responsibility

How responsible he is, to the limits of his capacity, for his own body, for his own safety. He holds his breath when a cloth covers his face. He widens his eyes in the dark. When he loses his balance, his hands curl around whatever comes under them, and he clutches the stuff of your shirt.

Within His Limits

How he is curious, to the limits of his understanding; how he attempts to approach what arouses his curiosity, to the limits of his motion; how he derives satisfaction from another face opposing itself to his face, to the limits of his attention; how he asserts his needs, to the limits of his force.

oo oo oo

RAE ARMANTROUT

Knowing You _____

You pull my face to yours until
the picture blurs.
New soul,
was this a funny thing
you wanted to show me?

*

That your small hand cups my cheek!
Classic gesture—
so unforeseeable.

*

You point at every truck and grunt;
I would rather watch the trees.

*

They design these
little cars to fill your diligent concern.
You align them on window sills,
crying when the last won't fit,
or turn them all wheel up
and raise your hands
in victory.

*

"What do you call what you're doing?"
is a question you dispense with.

*

Resolute,
in your smooth, dense flesh,
you finger torn cushions
and fuss.

oo oo oo

MAXINE CHERNOFF

How Lies Grow _____

The first time I lied to my baby, I told him that it was his face on the baby food jar. The second time I lied to my baby, I told him that he was the best baby in the world, that I hoped he'd never leave me. Of course I want him to leave me someday. I don't want him to become one of those fat shadows who live in their mother's houses watching game shows all day. The third time I lied to my baby I said, "Isn't she nice?" of the woman who'd caressed him in his carriage. She was old and ugly and had a disease. The fourth time I lied to my baby, I told him the truth, I thought. I told him how he'd have to leave me someday or risk becoming a man in a bow tie who eats macaroni on Fridays. I told him it was for the best, but then I thought, I want him to live with me forever. Someday he'll leave me: then what will I do?

oo oo oo

DIANE DI PRIMA

The Loba Sings to Her Cub _____

O my mole, sudden & perfect
golden gopher tunneling
to light, o separate(d)
strands of our breath!
                    Bright silver
threads of spirit
                O quicksilver
spurt of fist, scansion of
unfocussed eyeball,
                    grace of yr
cry, or song, my
cry or
        you lie warm,   wet on the
soggy pelt of my
                hollowed
belly, my
            bones curve up
to embrace you.

○○ ○○ ○○

BARBARA EINZIG

The Miracle of Tenses _____

She remembered it as a time of intense feeling, the days when their child had just been born. The child's amazement at being born was fully coincident with the event; the mother had never seen such an expression as was on her face. For her face was not used to being a face, to being seen; she had never been seen before. She was not amazed at something but in something, so she was not amazed at all, but was herself amazement. Then the baby slept, and the father slept, and she lay awake between them, because the baby had promised for so long to come that she must be prepared for waiting and then it was here. We are all here in the world where we are, but it had been somewhere else, and before that it had not been, so that despite the fact that we all have arrived here by being born, there is nothing more common, the event of the child's birth, the child's existence, was extraordinary, a paradox that did not escape her.

It was November, and the day of the naming ceremony it snowed. It was all white outside and the room was full of flowers. The snow did not last long, but melted cleanly in the strong sun, leaving no trace. Awake, the baby with her large dark eyes looked out the window and made graceful falling motions with her fists, remembering through these gestures where she had been and what she had been doing just before being born, but without thinking of that place or action as we do. The movements remembered themselves, they repeated themselves but now had space in which to fall and so, startling, they gradually forgot themselves and changed to open hands that learned to touch and hold.

Remembering this time puts it in the past, and it has been long enough ago now to want to do so, we want to live in the present moment. It hadn't been easy, and it seemed she couldn't just take or leave anything anymore, but had to worry about it and take care of it. Chains of tiny actions must be sustained: while being dressed, one hand keeps the baby from rolling off the changing table while the other dabs a washcloth into the warm water of a small bowl. Layers of clothing are resisted and go on with effort; all this must have been washed and prepared, in the middle knocked over, washed and soiled, it is washed and prepared and set out or put on again. At last they go out into the winter sunlight. While the leaves had been falling the baby had been

238

crying for her attention or squirming against her chest and even when it was asleep she was held to it in fascination. So when she looked up into the sky for the first time in a long time she saw the branches of sycamores and elms revealed—gray, white, chalky brown. Dark spots suspended among them were the nests of birds, and a squirrel ran easily out to where the branch thinned and bent under its nimble weight which, practiced, used this giving way as a springboard to the neighboring tree. The cool air makes the colors brittle, or the gold leaves are suddenly wasted, trunks further lined with shadows dark and defined where the branches that throw them are close by or soft shadows where the light is blocked further away.

The days turned into weeks that they counted its age by.

Remembering it put it in the past, though the power of the event continued to live in the form of the child and its life.

Is part of being in a new love remembering acts of this new love? And why does this remembering not put the act of love safely in the past but cause us to relive it as if it were a blood infusing us?

ALICIA OSTRIKER

from: Mother/Child _____

The door clicks. He returns to me.
He brings fresh air in.
We kiss, we touch. I am holding the flannel-wrapped baby.
The girls run to him.

He takes his jacket off and waltzes
the weightless
bundle over his shoulder.
We eat dinner, and evening falls.

I have bathed the girls. I walk by our broad bed.
Upon it rests a man
in a snow white shirt, like a great sleepy bird.
Next to him rests his seed, his son.

Lamplight falls on them both. If a woman looks, at such
a sight, is the felt pang
measureless pleasure?
Is it measureless pain?

oo oo oo

ANNE WALDMAN

To Baby ⸻⸻⸻⸻⸻⸻⸻⸻⸻

"A little Saint best fits a little shrine"

What you are makes me grow
younger to meet you.
Everything gets new,
lacks death. Heart
sighs "Beauty"
rocking lamb
to sleep.

While you cry, wind pauses
to learn the sound, then
applauds a loud lung.
You wear a dreamy
nightgown painted
clouds float
upon.

We all agree babies are
amazement. See, world,
how guileless & mild
is he. Smell every-
where Ivory Snow.
Hear him suck
tenderly.

What makes the cabin fresh?
Infant flesh! Huddled
against a tiny body,
a body doting
sings to you:

Rest your head my darling
Wee baby one
The stars are out
The canyon sleeps
Your life has just begun.

○○ ○○ ○○

ANNE WALDMAN

Baby's Pantoum ―――――――――――――――――

for Reed

I lie in my crib midday this is
    unusual I don't sleep really
Mamma's sweeping or else boiling water for tea
    Other sounds are creak of chair & floor, water
    dripping on heater from laundry, cat licking itself

Unusual I don't sleep really
    unless it's dark night everyone in bed
Other sounds are creak of chair & floor, water
dripping on heater from laundry, cat licking itself
    & occasional peck on typewriter, peck on my cheek

Unless it's dark night everyone in bed
    I'm wide awake hungry wet lonely thinking
occasional peck on typewriter, peck on my cheek
    My brain cells grow, I get bigger

I'm wide awake wet lonely hungry thinking
    Then Mamma pulls out breast, says "milky?"
My brain cells grow, I get bigger
    This is my first Christmas in the world

Mamma pulls out breast, says "milky?"
    Daddy conducts a walking tour of house
This is my first Christmas in the world
    I study knots in pine wood ceiling

Daddy conducts a walking tour of house
    I study pictures of The Madonna del Parto, a
    sweet-faced Buddha & Papago Indian girl
I study knots in pine wood ceiling
    I like contrasts, stripes, eyes & hairlines

I study pictures of The Madonna del Parto, a
sweet-faced Buddha & Papago Indian girl
    Life is colors, faces are moving

I like contrasts, stripes, eyes & hairlines
    I don't know what I look like

Life is colors, faces are moving
    They love me smiling
I don't know what I look like
        I try to speak of baby joys & pains

They love me smiling
    She takes me through a door, the wind howls
I try to speak of baby joys & pains
        I'm squinting, light cuts through my skin

She takes me through a door, the wind howls
    Furry shapes & large vehicles move close
I'm squinting, light cuts through my skin
        World is vast I'm in it with closed eyes

Furry shapes & large vehicles move close
    I rest between her breasts, she places me on dry leaves
World is vast I'm in it with closed eyes
        I'm locked in little dream, my fists are tight

I rest between her breasts, she places me on dry leaves
    He carries me gently on his chest & shoulder
I'm locked in little dream, my fists are tight
        They showed me moon in sky, was something
        in my dream

He carries me gently on his chest & shoulder
    He calls me sweet baby, good baby boy
They showed me moon in sky, was something
in my dream
        She is moving quickly & dropping things

He calls me sweet baby, good baby boy
    She sings hush go to sleep right now
She is moving quickly & dropping things
        They rock my cradle, they hold me tightly in their arms

She sings hush go to sleep right now
        She wears red nightgown, smells of spice & milk
They rock my cradle, they hold me tightly in their arms
        I don't know any of these words or things yet

She wears a red nightgown, smells of spice & milk
        He has something woolen and rough on
I don't know any of these words or things yet
        I sit in my chair & watch what moves

He has something woolen & rough on
        I can stretch & unfold as he holds me in the bath
I sit in my chair & watch what moves
        I see when things are static or they dance

I can stretch & unfold as he holds me in the bath
        Water is soft I came from water
I can see when things are static or they dance
        like flames, the cat pouncing, shadows or light
        streaming in

Water is soft I came from water
        Not that long ago I was inside her
like flames, the cat pouncing, shadows or light
streaming in
        I heard her voice then I remember now

Not that long ago I was inside her
        I lie in my crib midday this is
always changing, I am expanding toward you
        Mamma's sweeping or else boiling water for tea.

RACHEL BLAU DUPLESSIS

from: Tabula Rosa ————————————————————

House of the soul is filled with little
things, clay vessels, slipped and glazed
all smallness green leaf offering;
sweaty flower; baby loaf;
small as half an envelope which wads up tight
the poem's patchouli.

    . . .

Dabbles the blankie down
din
do throw foo foo
noo
dles the arror
of eros the error of arrows
each little spoil and spill
all during pieces fly apart.
Splatting crumb bits there and there.
Feed 'n' wipe. Woo woo petunia
pie.
Hard
to get the fail of it,
large small specks each naming
yellow surface
green bites
Red elbow kicks an orange tangerine.

The time inside, makes tracks, seems a small
room lurches into the foreground, anger, throwing, some
dash, power swirls up against MErock, pick it UP,
Mommy me NEED
it a push a touch a
putsch pull a flailing kick a spool
for her who is and makes thread
"I"
The she that makes her her
The she that makes me SHE

^.^

Practicing ferocity on $^{your}_{her}$ self

You become the mother   certainly a change.
           the monster   a chain.

     foaling
Is this failing the mother?
     finding

  ^.^

Top half poison   yellow light from above
ivy next half scritchings blue light swells from earth
the garden red   bruising a frame

      Digging, I sit on a flower.

Counting the steps of bright shadow, the pure pause, paces
clusters of ripe tones making up loud and then whispy forces
across one singular place saying no to itself with meditative
privation, yet unfixed, so spun out of, *or* of, being or
seeing. Which is not, but as it starts, starts a little
rivulet sound and voice, another, it fuses, pivots, a sigh
and sign; desire's design, blue transparencies rich for
thirst   listen, to listen is to drink
how can there be
another   cry: whom; one of another, who?
who cries? who listens?
hear here the liquid light
swirl and merge with drinking calls.
A sigh, a moan from what is waiting. Sweet sweet
sweet teas(e)
Another cry, a honey voice

Another
one.

  ^.^

All told, a voluminous backdrop:
crevices of the night, 4:32 exactly
silver hush behind, curdling
a shaggy hurt bleat.
Eat that moon's sweet light.
Bird's blood is brown.
Her words, some said, they're just a
"bandaid on a mummy."

Wad reams of rems into mâché
my eyes chewing.
She screams unassimilable
first dreams.

Hold her unutterable

And press another quire of girl bound in, bond in, for pink.
Draw drafts of "milk" these words
are milk the point of this is
drink.

oo oo oo

TILLIE OLSEN

from: *Yonnondio* _____

[Baby] Bess who has been fingering a fruit-jar lid—absently, heedlessly drops it—aimlessly groping across the table, reclaims it again. Lightning in her brain. She releases, grabs, releases, grabs. I can do. Bang! I did that. I can do. I! A look of neanderthal concentration is on her face. That noise! In triumphant, astounded joy she clashes the lid down. Bang, slam, whack. Release, grab, slam, bang, bang. Centuries of human drive work in her; human ecstasy of achievement, satisfaction deep and fundamental as sex: *I can do, I use my powers, I! I!* Wilder, madder, happier the bangs. The fetid fevered air rings with . . . Bess's toothless, triumphant crow. Heat misery, rash misery transcended.

oo oo oo

BOBBIE LOUISE HAWKINS

Them two little girls . . . _____

'Them two little girls was named Cora and Dora. They
was twins. They had an older sister . . . I don't remember what her
name was. That Cablet girl, Mama, that had the baby. . . .

'Miz Cablet would come down and she'd *talk* to Mama. She'd act so
mournful and so sad, and I finally caught on that it was this oldest girl
she was talking about. Finally this girl had a baby.

'Well, all this Miz Cablet would do would be to treat that girl like
she was dirt. She turned Mama against her. She turned us kids against
her.

'I told Mama, I said, Mama, I think that's real mean of Miz Cablet to
talk that way about her daughter. I said, I want to go down there and
see that baby!

'Mama said it was alright. So Hannah and me went down there and
here Cora and Dora was flitting around, you know. And the mother
was acting like she had a leper in her house. She was setting, the
daughter, was setting over in the corner in an old-fashioned rocker with
that tiny little baby. She just had her head bowed over it like this, you
know. She didn't even raise up her head when we come in.

'I went over and I told her, I said, We've come down here to see
your little baby. And she looked like she was so happy.

'It was the cutest little baby. I never could stand that woman after
that.'

BERNADETTE MAYER

Eve of Easter _____

Milton, who made his illiterate daughters
Read to him in five languages
Till they heard the news he would marry again
And said they would rather hear he was dead
Milton who turns even Paradise Lost
Into an autobiography, I have three
Babies tonight, all three are sleeping:
Rachel the great great great granddaughter
Of Herman Melville is asleep on the bed
Sophia and Marie are sleeping
Sophia namesake of the wives
Of Lewis Freedson the scholar and Nathaniel Hawthorne
Marie my mother's oldest name, these three girls
Resting in the dark, I made the lucent dark
I stole images from Milton to cure opacous gloom
To render the room an orb beneath this raucous
Moon of March, eclipsed only in daylight
Heavy breathing baby bodies
Daughters and descendants in the presence of
The great ones, Milton and Melville and Hawthorne,
          everyone is speaking
At once, I only looked at them all blended
Each half Semitic, of a race always at war
The rest of their inherited grace
From among Nordics, Germans and English,
          writers at peace
Rushing warring Jews into democracy when actually
Peace is at the window begging entrance
With the hordes in the midst of air
Too cold for this time of year,
Eve of Easter and the shocking resurrection idea
Some one baby stirs now, hungry for an egg
It's the Melville baby, going to make a fuss
The Melville one's sucking her fingers for solace
She makes a squealing noise
Hawthorne baby's still deeply asleep
The one like my mother's out like a light
The Melville one though the smallest wants the most

Because she doesn't really live here
Hawthorne will want to be nursed when she gets up
Melville sucked a bit and dozed back off
Now Hawthorne is moving around, she's the most hungry
Yet perhaps the most seduced by darkness in the room
I can hear Hawthorne, I know she's awake now
But will she stir, disturbing the placid sleep
Of Melville and insisting on waking us all
Meanwhile the rest of the people of Lenox
Drive up and down the street
Now Hawthorne wants to eat
They all see the light by which I write, Hawthorne sighs
The house is quiet, I hear Melville's toy
I've never changed the diaper of a boy
I think I'll go get Hawthorne and nurse her for the pleasure
Of cutting through darkness before her measured noise
Stimulates the boys, I'll cook a fish
Retain poise in the presence
Of heady descendants, stone-willed their fathers
Look at me and drink ink
I return a look to all the daughters and I wink
Eve of Easter, I've inherited this
Peaceful sleep of the children of men
Rachel, Sophia, Marie and again me
Bernadette, all heart I live, all head, all eye, all ear
I lost the prejudice of paradise
And wound up caring for the babies of these guys

oo oo oo

MARILYN HACKER

Third Snowfall _____

"Take with you also my curly-headed four-year-old child."
—*Josephine Miles: "Ten Dreamers in a Motel"*

Another storm, another blizzard
soaks the shanks and chills the gizzard.
Indoors, volumed to try a Stoic, a
four-year-old plays the *Eroica*
three times through. Young Ludwig's ears?
No, only an engineer's
delight in Running the Machine.
Pop! Silence? "I was just seein'
if I could make the tape run back."
"Don't." "If the knob is on 8-track
and I put on a record, what
happens? . . . It's turning, but it's not
playing." "That's what happens." "Oh.
Which dial is for the radio?
I'm going to jump up on your back!
Swing me around!" A subtle *crack*
and not-so-subtle knives-in-spine.
"Get down, my back's gone out! Don't whine
about it, I'm the one that's hurt."
"I'm sorry . . . Did I have dessert?
What's water made of? Can it melt?"
(I know how Clytemnestra felt.)
"I want a cookie. What is Greek?
Will I be taller by next week?
Is this the way a vampire growls?
I'm going to dress up in the towels.
Look! I can slide on them like skis!
Hey, I've got dried glue on my knees.
Hey, where are people from? The *first*
ones, I mean. What was the Worst
Thing you Ever Ate?" *Past* eight
at last, I see. "Iva, it's late."
"It's not. I want some jam on bread."
"One slice, then get your ass in bed."
"No, wait until my record's over.

I want my doll. And the Land Rover
for Adventure People. Mom, are
you *listening?* Where's the doll's pajamas?
There's glue or something in my hair.
Can I sleep in my underwear?
I think I need the toy fire-fighter
guy too ... I'm thirsty ..." *und so weiter.*

oo oo oo

ADRIENNE RICH

from: *Of Woman Born* _____

I remember one summer, living in a friend's house in Vermont. My husband was working abroad for several weeks, and my three sons—nine, seven, and five years old—and I dwelt for most of that time by ourselves. Without a male adult in the house, without any reason for schedules, naps, regular mealtimes, or early bedtimes so the two parents could talk, we fell into what I felt to be a delicious and sinful rhythm. It was a spell of unusually hot, clear weather, and we ate nearly all our meals outdoors, hand-to-mouth; we lived half-naked, stayed up to watch bats and stars and fireflies, read and told stories, slept late. I watched their slender little-boys' bodies grow brown, we washed in water warm from the garden hose lying in the sun, we lived like castaways on some island of mothers and children. At night they fell asleep without murmur and I stayed up reading and writing as I had when a student, till the early morning hours. I remember thinking: This is what living with children could be—without school hours, fixed routines, naps, the conflict of being both mother and wife with no room for being, simply, myself. Driving home once after midnight from a late drive-in movie, through the foxfire and stillness of a winding Vermont road, with three sleeping children in the back of the car, I felt wide awake, elated; we had broken together all the rules of bedtime, the night rules, rules I myself thought I had to observe in the city or become a "bad mother." We were conspirators, outlaws from the institution of motherhood; I felt enormously in charge of my life. Of course the institution closed down on us again, and my own mistrust of myself as a "good mother" returned, along with my resentment of the archetype. But I knew even then that I did not want my sons to act for me in the world, any more than I wished for them to kill or die for their country. I wanted to act, to live, in myself and to love them for their separate selves.

oo oo oo

SHARON OLDS

Pajamas

My daughter's pajamas lie on the floor
inside out, thin and wrinkled as
peeled skins of peaches when you ease the
whole skin off at once.
You can see where her waist emerged, and her legs,
her arms, and head, the fine material
gathered in rumples like skin the caterpillar
ramped out of and left to shrivel.
You can see, there at the center of the bottoms,
the raised cotton seam like the line
down the center of fruit, where the skin first splits
and curls back. You can almost see the hard
halves of her young buttocks, the precise
stem-mark of her sex. Her shed
skin shines at my feet, and in the air there is a
sharp fragrance like peach brandy—
the birth-room pungence of her released life.

SHARON OLDS

35/10 ─────────────────────────────

Brushing out my daughter's dark
silken hair before the mirror
I see the grey gleaming on my head,
the silver-haired servant behind her. Why is it
just as we begin to go
they begin to arrive, the fold in my neck
clarifying as the fine bones of her
hips sharpen? As my skin shows
its dry pitting, she opens like a small
pale flower on the tip of a cactus;
as my last chances to bear a child
are falling through my body, the duds among them,
her full purse of eggs, round and
firm as hard-boiled yolks, is about
to snap its clasp. I brush her tangled
fragrant hair at bedtime. It's an old
story—the oldest we have on our planet—
the story of replacement.

BESMILR BRIGHAM

from: House of the Lord, the Earth _____

will i forget my mother's hands

her face, to become a picture without

movement, the moment
photograph still in print, time of
sequence

her hand in my hand's drawing

not knowing what attachment is, or was—
find
her shape in dreams when i am old,
never more beautiful to me
than when death was on her, strange

her innocence

that i had never known or cared for, the
soft hair, wet with pain
sorrow
that she gave me knowledge for—she
had given her last rich gift, the circle
complete

alone, in herself
what she had believed did not matter; god
an abstraction, only that she had lived and was
dead
meant anything
        'i have lost my daughter' she
said. and 'i'm so glad you found me'
quick as a candle
burning low,
the voice

already broken, 'i was afraid i'd have to find you
—and i couldn't.' Oh she found me
(she found me) with such hurt
that glows each living thing; fast now
in secret places (interior)

       that only
sleep can bring

○○ ○○ ○○

SHERRIL JAFFE

Swing Low _____

Ann and Abraham were pushing the girls home from the school picnic. They had had a great time and so they had stayed too long and now they were overtired. They had ten blocks to go, and Lena was already starting to scream. Soon they would both be screaming. Ann started to sing: "Swing low, sweet chariot." Abraham joined her. He began to harmonize: "Comin' for to carry me home!" They sang the way parents have always sung to their children from the beginning of time—to lull them and soothe them and lift their spirits, to make their little lives like a musical comedy and, most of all, to drown them out.

oo oo oo

SHERRIL JAFFE

Something Larger ⸻⸻⸻⸻⸻⸻⸻

They spent minute after minute, hour after hour, year after year taking care of their children. Their children began helpless and needed everything done for them, but gradually they grew older and more self-reliant. Then they needed them less and less. Meanwhile, their parents had been growing older. Then their parents needed a little help, and then more and more. So they began to take care of their parents. They were tall and strong. Their energy was boundless. Then they themselves began to age. They didn't know what to make of it. They had always taken care of everybody else, now they needed someone to take care of them. They didn't want to admit it, they denied it. They didn't want to give in. But it didn't matter. Their children came to them and gathered round them. And finally they had to surrender. There was another presence in the room. Something larger.

oo   oo   oo

ACKNOWLEDGMENTS

Rae Armantrout: "Knowing You" printed by permission of the author.

Margaret Atwood: "Giving Birth" from *Dancing Girls* by Margaret Atwood. Copyright © 1977, 1982 by O. W. Toad, Ltd. Reprinted by permission of Simon & Schuster, Inc. and Jonathan Cape Ltd.

Carol Bergé: from *Acts of Love: An American Novel* (Bobbs-Merril, 1974). Copyright © 1974 by Carol Bergé. Reprinted by permission of the author.

Summer Brenner: "Spring Tide" and "Blissed Raga" from *From the Heart to the Center* (The Figures, 1977). Copyright © 1977 by Summer Brenner. Reprinted by permission of the author. "Whithertofore" and "Inches and Lives" from *The Soft Room* (The Figures, 1978). Copyright © 1978 by Summer Brenner. Reprinted by permission of the author. "Letter to an Unborn Daughter" printed by permission of the author.

Besmilr Brigham: from "House of the Lord, the Earth" printed by permission of the author.

Nicole Brossard: from *Journal intime*. Copyright © 1984 by Nicole Brossard. Reprinted by permission of the author and Les Editions de l'Hexagone. Translation copyright © 1989 by Lydia Davis.

Maxine Chernoff: "The Fetus" and "A Birth" from *Utopia TV Store* (Yellow Press, 1979). Copyright © 1979 by Maxine Chernoff. Reprinted by permission of the author. "How Lies Grow." Copyright © 1988 by Maxine Chernoff. Originally published in *American Poetry Since 1970: Up Late*, edited by Andrei Codrescu (Four Walls Eight Windows, 1988). Reprinted by permission of the author.

Laura Chester: "Who Knows" from *In the Zone: New and Selected Writings*. Copyright © 1988 by Laura Chester. Reprinted by permission of the author and Black Sparrow Press. "Suckle Sex," "Song of Being Born," and selection from "Primagravida" from *Primagravida* (Christopher's Books, 1975). Copyright © 1975 by Laura Chester. Reprinted by permission of the author. Two selections from *The Stone Baby*. Copyright © 1989 by Laura Chester. Reprinted by permission of the author and Black Sparrow Press.

Wanda Coleman: "Giving Birth" from *Imagoes*. Copyright © 1983 by Wanda Coleman. Reprinted by permission of the author and Black Sparrow Press.

Laurie Colwin: from *Another Marvelous Thing*, by Laurie Colwin. Copyright © 1982, 1983, 1984, 1985, 1986 by Laurie Colwin. Reprinted by permission of Alfred A. Knopf, Inc. and Donadio & Ashworth, Inc.

Lydia Davis: selections from "What You Learn" printed by permission of the author.

Toi Derricotte: selections from *Natural Birth* (The Crossing Press, 1983). Copyright © 1983 by Toi Derricotte. Reprinted by permission of the author.

Carole Itter: "Cry Baby" from *Whistle Daughter Whistle* (Caitlin Press, 1982). Copyright © 1982 by Carole Itter. Originally appeared in Fireweed. Reprinted by permission of the author.

Sherril Jaffe: "The Baby Laughs" and "Meanwhile, Back on Earth" from *The Unexamined Wife*. Copyright © 1983 by Sherril Jaffe. Reprinted by permission of the author and Black Sparrow Press. "Swing Low" and "Something Larger" from *The Faces Reappear*. Copyright © 1988 by Sherril Jaffe. Reprinted by permission of the author and Black Sparrow Press.

Frances Jaffer: selections from "Milk Song" from *Alternate Endings* (HOW[ever] Book Series, 1985). Copyright © 1985 by Frances Jaffer. Reprinted by permission of the author.

Erica Jong: "The Birth of the Water Baby" and "On the First Night" from *Ordinary Miracles* by Erica Jong. Copyright © 1983 by Erica Mann Jong. Reprinted by arrangement with NAL Penguin Inc., New York, New York and Sterling Lord Literistic.

Jane Lazarre: from *The Mother Knot* by Jane Lazarre (McGraw Hill Book Co., 1976). Copyright © 1976 by Jane Lazarre. Reprinted by permission of The Wendy Weil Agency, Inc., Virago Press Ltd. and David Higham Associates Ltd.

Lyn Lifshin: "North" originally appeared in *Leaning South*. Reprinted by permission of the author. "The Daughter I Don't Have" printed by permission of the author.

Joan Slesinger Logghe: "Madonna of the Peaches" and "Empty Breasts" printed by permission of the author.

Daphne Marlatt: two selections from "Rings" from *What Matters: Writing 1968-70* (Coach House Press, 1980). Copyright © 1980 by Daphne Marlatt. Reprinted by permission of the author.

Bernadette Mayer: two selections from *The Desires of Mothers to Please Others in Letters* printed by permission of the author. "Eve of Easter" printed by permission of the author.

Deena Metzger: from *Skin: Shadows/Silence* (West Coast Poetry Review, 1976). Copyright © 1976 by Daphne Marlatt. Reprinted by permission of the author.

Dea Trier Mørch: selections from *Winter's Child* by Dea Trier Mørch, translated by Joan Tate, reprinted by permission of the University of Nebraska Press. Copyright © 1976 by Dea Trier Mørch. Translation copyright © 1986 by Joan Tate.

Anaïs Nin: "Birth" from *Under a Glass Bell* by Anaïs Nin (Swallow Press, 1948). Copyright renewed 1976 by Anaïs Nin. All rights reserved. Reprinted by permission of The Author's Representative, Gunther Stuhlmann and Peter Owen Ltd.

Alice Notley: from *Songs for the Unborn Second Baby* (United Artists, 1979). Copyright © 1979 by Alice Notley. Reprinted by permission of the author.

Naomi Shihab Nye: "The Rattle of Wheels Toward the Rooms of the New Mothers" printed by permission of the author.

Joyce Carol Oates: "A Touch of the Flu," copyright © 1988 by The Ontario Review, Inc. From *The Assignation* published by The Ecco Press in 1988. Reprinted by permission.

Edna O'Brien: excerpt from *The Country Girls Trilogy* by Edna O'Brien. Copyright © 1960, 1962, 1964, 1986 by Edna O'Brien. Reprinted by permission of Farrar, Straus and Giroux, Inc. and George Weidenfeld & Nicolson Ltd.

Sharon Olds: "The Planned Child." Copyright © 1985 by Sharon Olds. Originally appeared in *Poetry*. Reprinted by permission of the author. "The Language of the Brag" reprinted from *Satan Says* by Sharon Olds by permission of the University of Pittsburgh Press. Copyright © 1980 by Sharon Olds. "The Moment," "Eggs," "New Mother," "Pajamas," and "35/10" from *The Dead and the Living* by Sharon Olds. Copyright © 1983 by Sharon Olds. Reprinted by permission of Alfred A. Knopf, Inc.

Tillie Olsen: from *Yonnondio* by Tillie Olsen. Copyright © 1974 by Tillie Olsen. Reprinted by permission of Delacorte Press/Seymour Lawrence, a division of Bantam, Doubleday, Dell Publishing Group, Inc.

Alicia Ostriker: "Propaganda Poem," "Letter to M.," and excerpt from "Mother/Child" from *The Mother/Child Papers* by Alicia Ostriker. Copyright © 1980 by Alicia Suskin Ostriker. Reprinted by permission of Beacon Press. "The Cambridge Afternoon Was Grey." Copyright © 1987 by Alicia Ostriker. Originally appeared in *Ploughshares*. Reprinted by permission of the author.

Jayne Anne Phillips: "Bluegill" from *Fast Lanes* by Jayne Anne Phillips. Copyright © 1987 by Jayne Anne Phillips. Reprinted by permission of the publisher, E. P. Dutton/Seymour Lawrence, a division of Penguin Books USA Inc.

Adrienne Rich: selection from "Mother and Son, Woman and Man" from *Of Woman Born, Motherhood as Experience and Institution*, by Adrienne Rich, is reprinted by permission of the author and W.W. Norton & Company, Inc. Copyright © 1986, 1976 by W.W. Norton & Company, Inc. Published in the U.K. by Virago Press Ltd. 1977.

Barbara Rosenthal: "Baby Moves Inside" from *Sensations* (Visual Studies Workshop Press, 1984). Copyright © 1984 by Barbara Rosenthal. Reprinted by permission of the author.

Miriam Sagan: "Armed Robbery" and "Heroines" printed by permission of the author.

Christine Schutt: "Sisters" printed by permission of the author.

Lynne Sharon Schwartz: from *Rough Strife* by Lynne Sharon Schwartz. Copyright © 1980 by Lynne Sharon Schwartz. Reprinted by permission of Harper & Row Publishers, Inc. and the Virginia Barber Literary Agency.

Arlene Stone: from "Son Sonnets" printed by permission of the author.

Sharon Thesen: "Elegy, The Fertility Specialist" originally appeared in *The Midnight Review*. Reprinted by permission of the author.

Joyce Thompson: "Dreams of a New Mother" from *East is West* by Joyce Thompson. Copyright © 1987 by Joyce Thompson. Reprinted by permission of Breitenbush Books.

With special thanks to my cousin, Penfield Chester, and to my editor, Betsy Uhrig. I would also like to thank Debbie Reed and Eric Wilska of the Bookloft in Great Barrington, Massachusetts.

Laura Chester, co-editor of *Rising Tides*, the first anthology of twentieth-century American women poets, was also one of the founding editors of the innovative small press, The Figures, as well as the editor of the anthology, *Deep Down: The New Sensual Writing by Women*. Over ten volumes of her poetry, fiction, and non-fiction have been published including, most recently, *Lupus Novice*, Station Hill Press; *Free Rein*, Burning Deck; *In the Zone: New & Selected Writing* and *The Stone Baby*, a novel, Black Sparrow Press. Laura Chester grew up in Wisconsin and has lived in New Mexico, Paris, and Berkeley. She now lives with her two sons in the Berkshires of Massachusetts, where she is planning a third anthology, *The Marriage Bed*, and working on a new collection of short fiction, *Bitches Ride Alone*.